Jaclyn's Journey

Dancing Through Life in Spite of Chronic Illness

By Lori Kaplan

Jaclyn's Journey

Dancing Through Life in Spite of Chronic Illness

Lori Kaplan

Published by:

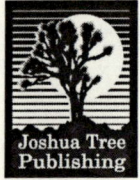 **Joshua Tree Publishing**

www.JoshuaTreePublishing.com

All rights reserved. No part of this book may be reproduced or transmitted in any form or by any means, electronic or mechanical, including photocopying, recording or by any information storage and retrieval system without written permission from the author.

Copyright © 2010 Lori Kaplan

ISBN: 0-9823703-9-3
13-Digit: 978-0-9823703-9-1

Printed in the United States of America

Dedication

To Alan and the amazing family
we have together—Jaclyn, Ryan and Joshua.

> For Linda --
> I hope you know how much Jaclyn enjoyed having you for a teacher. Thank you.
> Lori Kaplan

Acknowledgements

    I began this book as a gift to my daughter. I wanted her to know her story—all she had been through and how proud we were of her. In the process of writing, I realize how blessed I am to have so many amazing people in my life who have, in different ways, been on Jaclyn's Journey with her, with me, and with our family.

    Jaclyn, I'm so very glad to be your mom. Thanks, My Love, for being you, and for teaching me about dancing through life. I love how much you love me and how much I love you too. The thought of your smile, your laugh, and your hand in mine continues to light up my days. You will always be my sunshine. I love you...to the moon and back!

    To Ryan and Joshua, your spunk, spirit, intelligence, and creativity make me so proud. Thanks for giving me so much to laugh at and to love. You are, and will continue to be, bright sparkles in my life. I love being your mom!

    I am very fortunate to have an encouraging and supportive husband, Alan Silberman, who has shared this incredible journey with me. I'm so glad we have each other. Thanks for being so good at what you do, enabling me to be at home with our kids and sharing the day-to-day of their lives. I love you...more so than I ever imagined.

    I'm honored to have my mom, Judy Kaplan, play such a vital part in my life. YOU inspired ME to be a good mom. My kids are truly lucky to have you for their Mema. And, of course, your editing assistance is much appreciated.

I am very grateful to my brother, Danny Kaplan, for being such a fun-loving uncle to my kids, for his assistance in guiding me through this publication process, and most especially for the beautiful cover design he and his wife, Carrie Jardine, provided for my book.

I've been fortunate to have the support of many family members on this journey. A most special thank you to Karen and Alex Odishoo, Traci, Jennifer, and Michael Odishoo, Bernice Cobb, and Joan Davis for being so involved in my life and that of my family. I appreciate Corinne Odishoo for her outstanding work creating my website. Thank you to Bob and Roberta Silberman, Nancy Silberman, and all my in-laws and other family members as well. I hope each one of you knows how much you mean to my kids and to me as well.

I am indebted to the many friends who supported me in my role as Mom and Writer. A special thanks to Elaine Zemanek and Pauline Boss for reading early drafts and encouraging me to finish when it didn't seem possible. Your feedback and your friendship have meant the world to me. I am grateful to Jodie Johnson, Megan Juskiewicz, Diane Vilimek, Christie Wolf, Mena Lollino and Bill Allen for listening to Jaclyn's story many times and for occasionally whisking me away from it all. Thanks also to our school community and neighborhood for ongoing support.

A special acknowledgement to Dr. Ilbawi, Dr. Husayni, Dr. Barth, Dr. Joyce, Dr. Verges, Dr. Flynn, Dr. Lopata, and Dr. Zimmerman for taking excellent care of Jaclyn. Thanks to the many wonderful nurses we've grown to love over the years. I am also grateful to Cindy Jonker for medical editing.

John Paul Owles at Joshua Tree Publishing believed in Jaclyn's story and made this book a reality. I appreciate your guidance, competence, and assistance throughout this process. I am also grateful to my editor, Arlene, for all her time and patience as this book came together.

Thank you to all of Jaclyn's friends who journeyed with her and became such an important part of her life, and consequently my life as well. Memories of many of you dancing around our family room, doing crafts at our kitchen table, and playing games in our house will stay with me forever. To Bethany and Amber, you will always hold a special place in my heart because of your closeness to Jaclyn.

Table of Contents

Dedication	3
Acknowledgements	5
Table of Contents	7
Introduction	9
A Beautiful Baby Is Born	13
And Then the Bough Breaks	17
Learning the Ropes	23
Meeting the Surgeons	25
The Day of Surgery Arrives	29
More Bumps in the Road	33
You Know It's a Problem When…	41
Trying To Be "Normal"	43
Second Surgery is Scheduled	47
Therapies Begin	49
Just Being a Kid	53
Third Surgery: The Big One	57
Revising the Life Plan	63
She's a Regular Kid After All	67
It's Time to Start Doing Things Other People Do	71
Gearing Up For Round Four	75
"Normalcy" Sets in Yet Again	81
The Second Child Feels Like a First	89

Table of Contents (cont.)

My Needs Become Secondary	91
School Begins	95
An Extra Bonus Surgery	101
To Have or Not To Have a Third Child	105
Can't this Kid Catch a Break?	109
Hospital-Free Is a Good Way To Be	115
Being Different	135
Existing on the Fringe	143
Telling Jaclyn About Her Heart	147
Here We Go Again!	151
This Surgery Is Completely Different	159
Last-Minute Hassles	165
Fifth Open-Heart Surgery (and an Emergency Sixth!)	169
How Do You Thank Someone?	183
Not Letting Anything Stand in Her Way	187
Dessert Fest	191
Acclimating to Hospital Life	193
Sleeping and Eating at the Hospital	199
A Hospital is a Very Sad Place	201
The Things They Don't Tell You	205
How Do You Do It?	207
The Best Summer Ever	213
One Day	217
Jaclyn's Journey: Lessons She Taught Me	223
About the Author	227

Introduction

"Now remember, you might go home today without a baby," said the surgeon. And then with arms outstretched, he waited for us to hand him our precious child. He was ready to carry her into the operating room to try to fix her heart. She was six weeks old. I will never forget those words for the rest of my life. I can still hear the tone of his voice and feel the insensitivity of his comment. There was no way I wanted to hand my baby to him after hearing that, but I realized I had no choice.

That would be the first of many surgeries and procedures for my daughter, Jaclyn, who lives with Complex Congenital Heart Disease. By looking at her, no one could tell that she has endured more than anyone should ever have to. She has lived her life with hospitalizations, surgeries, procedures, medications, doctors' appointments, blood tests, medical equipment and adaptive therapies. Jaclyn knows no other way to live. She was 9 ½ years old when I began writing this book, and this is her journey. It is about her tremendous spunk and spirit, her ability to *dance through life* despite her heart condition, and her unwavering smile and perseverance in the face of adversity. This book is about the lessons she has taught me during her journey. It also touches on the experience of being Jaclyn's mother and how our family has endured living with chronic illness.

It has taken me 9 ½ years to start writing about this difficult journey. From the beginning, the day of Jaclyn's initial diagnosis at one month of age, friends, family, and colleagues all said the same thing: "write down your thoughts and feelings" as a way to "help you get through it." But back then I was concerned that Jaclyn would someday read about the feelings I was having: all my fears, all my worries, all we went through with this baby. I thought it would be better *not* to document these thoughts and feelings because they might someday scare her. I thought it would be better if she didn't have to know all that we lived through those first few years.

But it wasn't just those first few years that would be hard for Jaclyn and for us. When she was an infant, I told friends that I couldn't wait until she was three. Surgeons explained to us that by the age of three the "final repair" of her heart would probably be complete. I believed that after the final surgery we could begin a more "normal" life. We did not know, or perhaps naively could not have understood then, that we were embarking on a lifelong journey of what I have come to think of as "normal life" versus "the medical world." Fortunately, most of the time our family operates in "normal life" mode, but often "the medical world" creeps in, dominating or overpowering that normal life. This book is about how our family balances "normal life" versus "the medical world."

Another reason for my reluctance to write or journal when Jaclyn was a baby and toddler was because it served as a reminder of the person I used to be. Before I was Jaclyn's mom, I was a researcher, hoping to one day become a professor. I wrote scholarly articles about family caregiving during chronic illness. My work was published in peer-reviewed journals. I used to write research articles, book chapters, grants, and book reviews, but my life was changing before my eyes with my daughter's diagnosis of Complex Congenital Heart Disease. My days of working toward becoming a professor were numbered. Writing would only remind me of who I used to be, and I didn't want that memory.

So why have I finally documented Jaclyn's journey? I wish I had an answer. I still don't like the thought of putting down on paper my true feelings, concerns, and thoughts because they often *are* scary. But for some reason, the words are flowing out of me. Maybe it is therapeutic. Perhaps that is why in the middle of the night, when I can't sleep, I recall moments when Jaclyn was younger that I thought I had forgotten forever. Maybe now I can write about her journey because she has made it through so much already. When it was happening, it was simply too hard. Or maybe I am stronger now simply for having lived through some of these experiences. I take pride in acknowledging that we have, indeed, made it through a lot. We have packed a lot into Jaclyn's years, and we have not just "survived." Even though it is difficult at times, I think we have somehow thrived! Jaclyn has endured so much, yet always with a smile on her face, a contagious giggle from the bottom of her toes, and a dance in her step! Maybe other families who live with chronic illness, or even those who do not, can take something from our journey…from Jaclyn's journey.

A Beautiful Baby Is Born

My husband, Alan, and I dated in college, and after a long-distance relationship over eight years, we married. He was on track for success in the computer industry while I was completing my Ph.D. in Family Social Science at the University of Minnesota. My research interests focused on spousal caregiving to a mate with Alzheimer's Disease. I could cite every research article that had been written about caregiving during chronic illness.

When I got my degree, we moved to Chicago. On the day of our fourth anniversary, I found out I was pregnant. I spent the day relishing my secret. I couldn't wait to tell Alan in person when he came home from work. I remember having eaten lunch with my grandmother and cousin that day and smiling because I had a baby growing inside me that nobody knew about. I bought an anniversary card for Alan and inside I wrote "You're going to be a Daddy!" He came home from work that evening, put his computer bag away, found the card resting on a huge teddy bear, and he grinned from ear to ear. We went to dinner to celebrate both our anniversary and our pregnancy. We talked and planned. I brainstormed baby names. He thought of items we would have to purchase. We both realized our apartment would not be big enough for our growing family. We were very excited!

I remember people's reactions when we told them we were going to have a baby. There was lots of guessing about whether it would be a boy or a girl. Looking back, there were also remarks like, "doesn't matter—just so long as it's healthy." Who knew then that those comments would still echo in my ears? Does that mean people would love my child less because she was born with heart anomalies? Certainly not, but those comments still play around in my head.

I secretly wanted a little girl more than I could imagine. I always wanted two children, one boy and one girl, but I dreamed of having a girl first. I am the oldest girl in my family with a younger brother. Everyone we knew with children had girls, so we figured that statistically we were destined for a boy this first time.

My pregnancy was normal and easy. I was healthy. I underwent regular ultrasounds, and all was fine. My mom, who lived in California at the time, could not wait to be a grandmother, my grandmother was very excited to be a first-time great-grandmother, and my in-laws were excited too. My mom flew into town the week before I was due because she did not want to miss the birth of her first grandchild.

During the time I was pregnant with Jaclyn, Elton John had a hit song called *Blessed*. The first time I heard the song on the radio, I had to pull over in my car because I was crying so hard. It was as if Elton John was singing about my baby and the life we were going to have! It was a beautiful song about a child not yet born who was already so loved and so blessed. The words were everything I had felt for the child I was carrying inside me. I knew that Alan and I, as well as our families, would love this child to the ends of the earth. The song ends with a promise that "you'll have the best" and that "you'll be blessed." For the last few months of my pregnancy, that was my child's theme song.

Jaclyn was born on her due date, May 6, 1996. When the doctor said it was a girl, I remember being shocked. I can still hear myself asking, "It's a girl? It's a girl?" Then I held that amazing 6 lb. 11 oz. baby with a head full of black hair, and I was in love. She was beautiful and perfect in every way!

After two days in the hospital with our new baby, there was no hint anything was out of the ordinary. When the pediatrician came to check Jaclyn once more before we were discharged, she heard a slight heart murmur. My mom reported that as an infant I had a benign murmur. The pediatrician did not seem worried, but she paged a cardiologist "just to be sure." This doctor concurred that

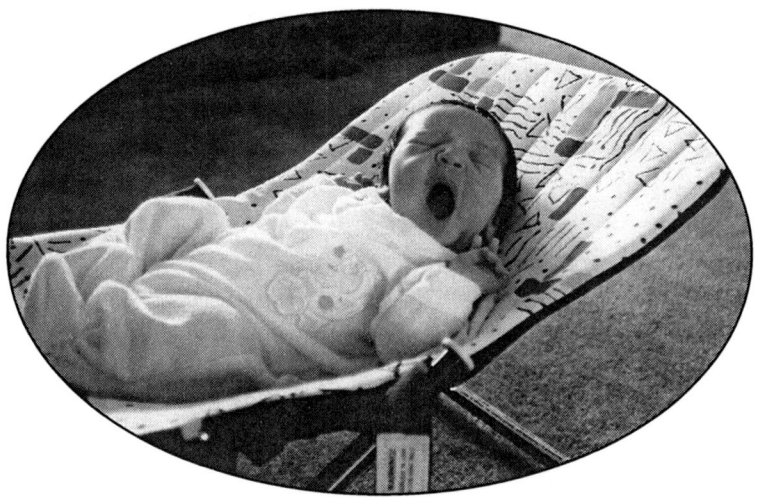

Jaclyn at one week of age, May, 1996.

it was most likely a benign murmur that would disappear on its own, "probably within a month" we were told. We scheduled a follow-up cardiology visit for one month later. How could we know that this next appointment would be a life-altering moment for all of us?

We took Jaclyn home without any idea of what future lay ahead for her or for us. At her one week check-up at the pediatrician's office, I asked why Jaclyn slept so much, especially right after eating. I was assured that many babies fall asleep while nursing and not to be concerned. By the second week, I had to ask the pediatrician for tips on how to wake Jaclyn because she was not waking on her own to eat. The nurses commented that I was lucky to have a baby who slept so much. But because she was a bit jaundiced at birth, I was reminded to be sure she ate on schedule. Waking her to eat was becoming more and more difficult. She simply wanted to sleep—a lot!

Being a nervous first-time mother, I brought Jaclyn back to the pediatrician when she was three weeks old because I was concerned about how she looked when she was breathing. Every time she took a breath, I noticed an indentation between her chest and abdomen. It looked like she was working hard to breath, and it made me nervous. The pediatrician said that it was just "immature chest development" and that, again, many babies are born this way. "Not to worry," I was told. "She'll grow, and all will fix itself," said the pediatrician.

Just shy of her four-week birthday, we held a baby naming and open house for Jaclyn. After the temple ceremony, our relatives and friends came to our home to see our precious girl. The day after the party, my mom left Chicago for her home in California. She had been living with us for a month, helping with her first grandchild. That afternoon I made a cassette tape of songs for Jaclyn. The first song on the tape was Elton John's *Blessed*. The rest of the songs were about things I wished for her, songs about my love for her, and songs about my dreams for her. I haven't been able to listen to the tape since the weekend I made it.

Lessons Jaclyn Taught Me.

If there's something you don't understand, ask! During Jaclyn's first few weeks of life, I had concerns. I insisted on bringing her to the pediatrician multiple times to be sure everything was all right. They assured me she was fine. My concerns persisted and so did my nagging questions to the doctors. With a newborn, I was learning the importance of asking questions and voicing my concerns when they arose. I didn't know then that life with Jaclyn would always entail extra vigilance, but looking back I realize I learned it soon after she was born.

And Then the Bough Breaks

Monday, June 3, 1996. Why do I remember the day? First of all, it was my mother's birthday. Second, it was supposed to be my husband's first day back at work after four weeks of paternity leave. However, as luck had it, he chose to work at home that day. This was the day I had scheduled Jaclyn's one month check-up with the cardiologist, the day the cardiologist was supposed to tell us the benign murmur was gone and to have a nice life, the day that was supposed to be the last time we ever had to see a pediatric cardiologist again.

Although Alan was supposed to be "working at home," I convinced him to come with me to the appointment with the pediatric cardiologist. We sat in the Pediatric Subspecialties waiting room holding Jaclyn. Looking around, there were families of children with all kinds of disabilities—obvious physical impairments and cognitive disabilities as well. When I was a college student, I worked with disabled children, and during graduate training, I had spent much time observing and interviewing impaired elders in nursing homes. I was not unfamiliar with disability, and I had studied family relationships in the face of illness. However, in that "subspecialties" waiting room, I whispered to Alan that we were lucky to have a healthy child. I was glad we would never have to come to this place again.

They called our name. We went into a little room with a half-circle couch, an examining table, a chair, and a desk. A big machine was wheeled in. It was an echocardiogram machine to take Jaclyn's first ultrasound. We lay her on the table and relaxed as the technician began the exam.

Neither Alan nor I were nervous about this appointment. After all, we had a perfect life! We had just bought our first house. We had family who loved us. We had many friends. Alan had a great job at Microsoft. I had completed my first year of a prestigious post-doctoral fellowship at the University of Chicago. My schedule was flexible enough to allow me to take three or four months off to stay home with Jaclyn and then to work part-time while she was in daycare. I was going places. I was publishing papers. I was teaching classes at the University of Chicago—my dream job and a fabulous university. We had a brand-new, happy, gorgeous baby girl. All our dreams were in place.

The technician seemed to be taking a very long time to finish this ultrasound. She was rubbing gel on our daughter's chest, moving a probe back and forth, while looking at images on a screen. My husband and I watched the screen but had no idea what we were looking at. There were colored globs, swishing to and fro as the technician moved the probe. Red, yellow, green, blue. I wasn't really worried about it so I paid little attention. But Alan was watching.

After what seemed like forever, the technician got up and left the room. She informed us that the cardiologist would review the tapes and be in to talk to us. We waited and waited. *Why was this taking so long?* I wondered. Finally, a doctor came in and introduced himself to us. He was not the same cardiologist who had seen Jaclyn after she was born. This doctor, who had reviewed the ultrasound, now picked up the probe and began moving it around Jaclyn's chest himself. He sat with his back to us, looking at the screen. We still did not know what he could see on the screen of colored blobs that would change our lives forever.

Finally, the cardiologist turned his chair around and spoke. I remember only a few select words and phrases from that day. The easy words, the comprehensible parts of the diagnosis: "Missing the pulmonary artery." "Hole in her heart." "Needs to be repaired." It was the more technical explanation from that day that I either didn't hear, didn't understand, or perhaps blocked out. I remember seeing tears stream down Alan's face. I didn't cry though. I was thinking that a hole in the heart was no big deal. Our friend's daughter had a hole in her heart, and it was easily repaired surgically. She was fine. Looking at my daughter, who appeared to be perfectly okay, I could only surmise that she'd be fine too. The rest of the words the cardiologist was uttering weren't registering for me: "Pulmonary atresia." "Transposition of the great arteries." "Complete AV septal defect." "Multiple aortic pulmonary collateral arteries." All I understood was that we had hit a minor bump in the road. I thought my daughter would need a small surgery to fix a hole, and that would be that. End of story. End of cardiology visits.

Then, suddenly, the doctor opened the door and told an assistant to call the intensive care unit (ICU) of the pediatric hospital. He wanted a bed prepped for Jaclyn. She was going to be admitted to ICU! I was confused. I heard him say Jaclyn was in congestive heart failure. I was thinking: *There must be a mistake. Look at her. She's fine. How can she be in congestive heart failure?* I didn't understand what was happening. Even if she needed surgery to fix a hole in her heart, what was all the fuss? Those surgeries were relatively common in the 1990s. Tears were still coming down my husband's face. I, however, was not processing all that was happening around me.

The doctor left us alone in that tiny room with the orange, purple and fuschia print couch. He told us it might take some time for the ICU to prepare a bed. We were to wait until the bed was ready and then walk Jaclyn down the long hallway connecting the doctors' office building to the hospital. The long hallway separating children who are having check-ups from those who are in ICU with something more serious than what a doctor can fix in an office.

We sat in that room with Jaclyn for a long time. At first we didn't speak at all, we just held our baby, stroking her full head of hair and looking into her big, navy blue-colored eyes. Then my husband started talking, and the more he talked, the angrier I got. He was connecting the dots for me regarding the cardiologist's words. It was sinking in. *Jaclyn is very sick. Jaclyn needs surgery. Jaclyn isn't coming home with us today because she is being admitted to the intensive care unit. Jaclyn is missing pieces of her heart. They just didn't grow.*

How could this be? I thought. *How could a baby who seemed so healthy, who was always so happy, and who was so easy to care for, be as sick as they were making her out to be?* It just did not make sense.

The longer we sat there, the more I started *hearing* the words.

At some point, I realized the transformation we were about to make. The "family with healthy child" label no longer fit us. We now were a "couple with a chronically sick child. A very sick child." My head started focusing on research articles about chronic illness. I started realizing what this diagnosis meant: that our lives would never be the same again; that the goals and plans we had for Jaclyn might not ever be realized; and that once we walked out the door of that stupid little room our lives would forever be changed. Our dreams were being shattered.

Staying in that room was somehow comforting. It was the last place Jaclyn, Mom and Dad had been while still that "family with a healthy child." Once we walked out of that room, once we journeyed down that long corridor to the hospital, our label changed. Ours was about to become one of the families I had studied. I was about to become a "caregiver" to a sick child, instead of just a "mommy." What I knew from text books and research articles was that chronic illness in the family isn't fun. Boy, how I wished at that moment that I had studied anything that didn't have to do with family relationships! Right at that moment, I didn't want to know what all the research said about families living with illness.

Later, we were asked if we wanted to call anyone. My first thought was that I couldn't call my mom. It was her birthday, and she had only been back in California for less than a day. She had just left us, and everything was fine. How could I call her and tell her that her granddaughter was very sick? I didn't want to do it.

Alan called his family and tried to get the words out but couldn't. I remember that he dropped the phone because he became hysterical. My in-laws and my aunt and uncle rushed to the hospital, and my mom caught a flight and arrived later that evening.

By then, we had made that terrible journey down the hall to the hospital. Jaclyn was put into an ICU bed. It was a room that was shared by three children. I hated it. It was filled with monitors, IV poles, and cribs with high rails so you couldn't reach in to touch your child easily.

Nurses came in and out. Jaclyn was undressed. Her adorable little clothes were put into a sterile, plastic bag and stuffed under the hospital bed. She wouldn't need those for a while. She was dressed in hospital clothes. She was weighed and measured. IVs were administered. Jaclyn cried. Monitors were hooked up. They beeped incessantly. Different people kept asking us the same questions over and over. "Was the pregnancy normal?" "Were there any complications?" "How is your own health?" "Your husband's health?" "Your parents' health?" "Did any family members have heart problems?" It went on and on. We answered all the questions, we stepped aside, we didn't hold our baby when she cried because she was in a hospital bed surrounded by multiple doctors and nurses. We were too shocked to even ask questions.

We stayed in that ICU room, hour after hour, watching the monitors. Numbers went up. Then they went down. For a long time I didn't even know what I was looking at. Monitors are filled with numbers. Heart rate. Respirations. Oxygen levels. Blood pressure. I didn't know what the numbers were supposed to be, so I truly had no idea how far off Jaclyn's numbers were. But I sat vigilantly and watched those numbers because that's what everybody seemed to be doing.

At some point I remember a rush of questions coming to my mind. I wanted to know how this happened. *What had we done? What had I done?* The doctor who was with us in that damn little room in Pediatric Subspecialties had come to answer our questions. He began by telling us that this was not our fault. That Jaclyn's heart anomalies were a "fluke of nature." That nothing we did caused it, and that it wasn't genetic. This man, this man whom I barely knew, whom I didn't want to know, was becoming a lifeline of information. We have since spent 9 ½ years seeing him regularly, and he has become like a member of our family.

Lessons Jaclyn Taught Me.

What's on the inside isn't necessarily what you see on the outside. Jaclyn's complex cardiac anomalies weren't visible to strangers. Nobody could ever tell by looking at her, even as a baby, that her heart didn't develop the way it was supposed to. The seriousness of her cardiac condition was not reflected by the happy, easygoing, pleasant and bright newborn, toddler and then grade-school child that Jaclyn was to become. We didn't try to hide her condition, but rather she just never acted like a sick child—and consequently we didn't treat her like one. I think that served her well.

Learning the Ropes

There is no privacy in an ICU room. Eventually I realized I hadn't nursed Jaclyn in hours. In all the shock and chaos of the afternoon turning into evening, it dawned on me that my baby hadn't eaten! I was encouraged to nurse her. So there I sat, with a towel draped over me, trying to nurse a baby who now had tubes and wires attached to her body in more places than I cared to imagine. I didn't know how to hold her. I didn't want to pull any wires that I shouldn't. I didn't want to hurt her. It felt awful. And I was scared.

Sometime during the next day or so, it was decided that nursing was too strenuous for Jaclyn; it was causing her to burn too many calories. But the doctors wanted her to have the breast milk for nourishment. That's when "The Pump" entered my life. The first few times I had to use a pump to extract my breast milk, it was excruciatingly painful. I sat in a chair, holding two funnels to my breasts. With the flick of a switch, this machine sucked the milk out of me and into bottles. Tears of pain mixed with tears of anger and frustration. But despite the pain, I wanted her to have the breast milk, so I pumped and I pumped. I was saddened to be denied the nursing experience I had so enjoyed with my daughter.

I don't remember all the details of those first few days. I do remember our families forcing Alan and me to leave the hospital at some point to go home and shower. We hadn't been home in several days and didn't realize how nice our own shower and towels really were. We had, instead, been taking turns sleeping down the hall from the ICU on chairs that folded out to become beds. These chairs were uncomfortable and not as clean as we would have liked. However, after a few sleepless days and nights, lying down at all simply felt good.

We also learned during those first days in ICU that other babies seemed to have little contact with anyone other than nurses and doctors. There was a newborn sharing the ICU room with Jaclyn. It was days before we ever saw a visitor for this child. He cried. Nurses tried to comfort him if they happened to be in the room at the time. But other times Alan and I, or our family members, were the only ones to hear this poor child scream. After hours of this, my mom asked the nurses if she could hold and comfort him. Of course, the answer was "no," but it was heartbreaking to hear and watch him squirm in his bed with no one close by.

I do not mean to be judgmental, but at the time I was wondering *Where are the parents?* I recognize that we have insurance, and that my husband and I can take time off from work, indefinitely when need be, to spend time with our child in the hospital. I also recognize that we have family who, near or far, are there for us. I have seen infants, toddlers, and young children over the years, alone in hospitals. At night, after work, or on weekends, the parents come. We, on the other hand, never leave. For us, there is simply no life away from the hospital while Jaclyn is there.

Meeting the Surgeons

During that first week in ICU, Jaclyn underwent a cardiac catheterization. The goal of this procedure, performed by the cardiologist, was to determine whether fixing her heart was even possible. A catheter was inserted into an artery in her groin and was fished up toward her heart to take pictures and measurements of pressures inside her arteries. I told myself over and over again: *Of course it would be possible to fix Jaclyn's heart. How could it not be?* I reasoned that it just *had* to be possible because I could not see it turning out any other way.

The day of the catheterization, Alan and I went outside for some fresh air. I needed it to be a bright, sunny day. To me, sunshine would mean that the catheterization would go well and that fixing her heart was doable. I didn't care what else they had to say when they were done with the procedure, except to tell us her heart could be repaired. When we went outside, it was cloudy. I started to cry.

The procedure took a few hours. When it ended, an assistant came running outside to tell us three things: (1) it was over; (2) Jaclyn was okay; and (3) fixing her heart was doable. Prayer number one answered! It was time to meet the surgeons.

We were told there were two surgeons who would perform Jaclyn's first surgery. We needed to meet them both and have the whole procedure explained to us. One surgeon was on-staff at the hospital where we were. We met him first.

On the day of this consultation, both of our families piled into a room. There sat the surgeon, upright and stiff. He drew heart diagrams and passed them across the table for us to see. He explained what he needed to do. He answered questions. He talked about the complexities of our daughter's anatomy in a stoic manner.

Apparently, I offended this Man of Greatness. I asked him how often he had performed *this* surgery before. His answer was that this combination of anomalies was rare, "maybe 1 in 10,000." I asked if he felt he could do it. He brushed me off with an arrogant comment along the lines of "how dare you ask me that question." He had a condescending attitude and poor people skills. Then I asked to see his hands. I don't know why I asked this, but it was important to me to see the hands of the man who would work on my daughter's heart. He thought I was a nut. He never showed me his hands.

This Man of Greatness rattled off terminology about the type of surgery to be performed. "Unifocalization of the left arteries." A few months later, "unifocalization of the right arteries." "A Rastelli." "Closing of the AV septal defect." This was my child we were talking about. There he sat rattling off the names of other surgeons who had perfected procedures. I asked if *this* surgery was so rare that it could be named after him upon completion. I don't know why I thought of this. But it came across as if he thought completion of this procedure would put his name in the medical books. So I asked. Instead of answering my question, he stood up with a look of contempt for me. I didn't mean disrespect, but rather I just wanted to know how rare this really was, and if he truly believed he could do it. Maybe my words came out wrong, but I simply wanted to know more. There were no bones about it; I despised this man.

Two days later we went to meet the other surgeon. He was not on staff at the hospital where we were, but he had privileges to perform surgeries there. We had been told that this man was the "best in the Midwest" and that he traveled all over to perform pediatric cardiac surgeries. His hospital was an hour away. Driving there and meeting him was the longest we had been away from Jaclyn. Our families stayed with her in her ICU room.

From the moment we met this surgeon, from the first time he shook Alan's hand and stroked my hand, I knew this man was wonderful. He sat down with us and very gently explained what needed to be done to repair Jaclyn's heart. Jaclyn was born with Complex Congenital Heart Disease. She had pulmonary atresia, which means her pulmonary artery, the main artery from her heart to her lungs, was missing. She also had transposition of the great arteries. The aorta, and what was supposed to be her pulmonary artery, were reversed. Third, she had a hole in her heart. Some holes are atrial (between the upper two chambers of the heart) and some are in the lower chambers of the heart (ventricular). Jaclyn's hole was rather large and was both atrial and ventricular. Finally, she had multiple aortic pulmonary collateral arteries (MAPCAs). To compensate for not having a pulmonary artery, her body grew tiny vessels to get blood from her aorta to her lungs. These vessels were what kept her alive. However, there were so many of them, and they were so small, that they would not sustain her indefinitely. She would outgrow them. They needed to be "unifocalized" which meant combined into one larger artery on each side of her heart and given a common origin.

This surgeon, after explaining in detail her diagnosis to us, also drew heart diagrams. But his were different. He drew upside down, so while we sat across from him at a table, we could see what he was drawing. The ease and grace with which he drew an upside-down heart, with all its anatomical parts, relaxed me. He was comforting and kind. He was calming. He answered every single question we had. I asked him if I could see his hands. He lay them on the table, outstretched for me to see. First he turned them palm-side up for me to look at, then he turned them over, ever so gracefully, so I could see them, palm-side down. He took his time as if this wasn't **THE MOST RIDICULOUS** thing any parent had ever asked him. I knew I wanted him to be Jaclyn's surgeon.

During the ride back to the ICU, I told my husband I did not want the first surgeon anywhere near Jaclyn. However, I knew that both surgeons would work together and deep down I was pleased that the "best in the Midwest" would take the lead over the first surgeon whom I had detested. Alan's question to me was, "Why does a surgeon have to be nice, if he's good at what he does?" I responded, "Why is it so much to ask that a surgeon be both? Shouldn't I want one who is both excellent at his craft and also humane?"

After one week in ICU in congestive heart failure, Jaclyn was stabilized and ready to go home. We were given prescriptions for various heart medications. We knew that fixing her heart was doable, and we knew that surgery was scheduled in ten days. We went home to try to be "normal."

The Day of Surgery Arrives

Jaclyn was now six weeks old. It had been two weeks since she was discharged from the hospital. The night before her first surgery, I gave her a bath and found myself transfixed by her naked little body. I knew this was the last night she would ever be scar-free. Tears welled up in my eyes as I imagined a surgeon cutting open her skin and creating permanent scars.

It had been explained to us that the incision for the unifocalization of her arteries would be made under her left arm pit, horizontally, going toward her back. We were told the surgeons had to cut through muscle, which meant physical therapy would be required later to regain strength. The first of many surgeries was about to begin. The unifocalization would join the tiny MAPCA arteries together, giving them a common origin on the left side of her heart. She would need the same thing done on the right side a few months later.

Bright and early on the day of surgery, we drove Jaclyn to the hospital. We were put into a surgical recovery room—a misnomer, because it's not really a room. It's a bed and a chair with curtains separating one family or patient from the next. People wait here until they are wheeled into surgery. Again, there is really no privacy.

Jaclyn was undressed. Consent forms were read and signed. The anesthesiologist came to meet us. Then we waited for the surgeons. Only the first surgeon came in that time, the one I disliked, while the other was en route to the hospital. Although it had only been ten days since we had met both surgeons, heard the details of the surgery, and discussed the risks involved, we had obviously had some time to go home and think about this. We had some idea of what to expect.

We were ready to go—as ready as any parent could be on the day his/her child needs surgery. Here we were, with the first surgeon, this cold man, standing in the surgical recovery room. He did not look at or touch Jaclyn, and she was right there in our arms! He had never seen her before. He had only met Alan and me the previous week. Then he uttered those words that will live inside my head forever: "Now remember, you might go home today without a baby." Trembling, I wondered, *what kind of a person says something like that just moments before surgery is to begin?* We clutched Jaclyn one more time, hugged her with such intensity, and cried so hard that neither of us could see clearly. Then the surgeon took Jaclyn and walked with her into the operating room. We were left standing outside the operating room as the door automatically shut. We hugged. We cried. We did not move for a long time.

The surgery took several hours. We sat in the surgical waiting room with family members close by. When it was over, both of the surgeons told us all had gone well, Jaclyn was fine, and we could see her soon.

I had no idea what to expect when we walked into the ICU that first time. Jaclyn was lying on her side in the bed, propped by pillows. There were numerous wires attached to different parts of her body. But what I noticed most of all was that this baby didn't look like my beautiful Jaclyn at all. She had a large bandage over the incision sight, under her left armpit. There was dried blood all around it. Then I saw a tube sticking out of her body, a chest tube an inch or so below the incision, a second scar. Having never had surgery myself, nor ever having seen someone so soon after surgery, I had no reference point for chest tubes or draining fluids. Seeing a tube sticking out of my tiny six-week old made me cringe. It would be the first of many times I felt sick to my stomach.

There was also a ventilator and a big tube coming out of Jaclyn's mouth, taped to her lips and cheek. This tube was connected to a machine that breathed for her. It was loud, and it frightened me.

Later that afternoon, the cardiologist and the surgeon I liked checked on Jaclyn numerous times. This surgeon, the one who was not even in his own hospital, the one who drove an hour to perform this procedure, the one who so graciously showed me his hands, came in to Jaclyn's ICU room and stroked her hair. He rubbed her side and sat down to see if we had any questions. He treated her like a person, a baby, and knew how to speak to us as parents.

Needless to say, the other surgeon, over the course of our two-week stay in ICU in *his* hospital, poked his head into Jaclyn's room only once. He stood in the doorway, asked how she was doing, and left. He never took the time to walk fully into the room, to gaze at her in the bed, to see Jaclyn as the baby we loved. This was not his style, and I continued to fault him for it in my mind.

Jaclyn spent two weeks in the hospital recovering from surgery. She would need oxygen at home while her lungs healed. In the six weeks since she was diagnosed, we learned more cardiac anatomy than either of us had ever cared to know. We also learned what was "normal" for Jaclyn and when to really panic. There was one more thing for us to learn before we were discharged from the hospital: cardio pulmonary resuscitation (CPR). While it is certainly not bad for anyone to learn or re-learn CPR, it was not comforting to know that we were being taught how to perform this procedure on Jaclyn.

And then we were sent home.

More Bumps in the Road

When Jaclyn was discharged from the hospital, she required medical equipment. In addition to a few more medications, an oximeter was delivered to our home. We attached this machine to Jaclyn's toe in order to monitor her oxygen levels and heart rate. At first we kept the oximeter on her foot, day and night. As she got older, we referred to the oximeter as her *E.T. light* because the sensor that wraps around a finger or toe emits a red spark of light, like the alien in the Steven Spielberg movie. The machine displayed readings, and alarms sounded when Jaclyn's oxygen levels or heart rate dropped below a set rate. Jaclyn set off the alarm all the time.

Normal oxygen levels for the majority of the population are close to 100. As an infant, Jaclyn's oxygen level varied anywhere from the upper 70s to upper 80s. When she cried, her oxygen level would drop. She would become rather blue around her lips and on her fingertips. When she stopped crying, her numbers would slowly climb back up. In the ICU, new nurses who hadn't yet cared for Jaclyn became nervous when her numbers were all over the chart! By the time we had been in ICU for two weeks, we had become familiar with her "normal."

Living with an oximeter at home definitely took its toll. Not only would Jaclyn's numbers drop when she cried, but the monitor was also sensitive to movement. During the daytime this was not much of an issue because we could see that despite alarm bells ringing, Jaclyn was okay. After a few weeks, we stopped using the machine during the day. And after weeks of oxygen at home, we were able to gradually wean her from that as well.

    Nighttime was a different story. Every time Jaclyn's numbers would drop, every time she would turn over or move in her sleep, the alarms went off. My husband and I would race to her bedroom, shine a mini flashlight onto her face to see if she was blue, and then mute the alarm. For the first few weeks, we would both panic every time alarms rang, and both of us would run to her room. Sometimes we could sleep a few hours without hearing the alarm. Other times it would beep every few minutes. While she was never in distress, we continued racing to her room, deliriously sleep-deprived, just to be sure. After weeks of this, we started to accept that she was, indeed, all right. Eventually we took turns clamoring to her bedroom, one of us rolling over to remind the other that it was not our turn to go. This is what sleep deprivation does to adults.

    On many occasions I slept on Jaclyn's bedroom floor with my hand on the oximeter's reset button. I was overcome with exhaustion, and this was easier than going back and forth between her room and mine. It took months before we felt brazen enough to eliminate nightly use of the oximeter, except for occasional checks of her levels or when she was sick.

    After the first surgery, my mom had stayed to help care for Jaclyn. There were little things I could not do alone while Alan was at work. For instance, I couldn't take Jaclyn in the car by myself. Her head would flop down in the car seat, as all two to three month olds do, but for her this made breathing difficult. So in order for her to ride in the car, somebody had to sit in the back seat and hold her chin and head up while we drove. Jaclyn had numerous follow-up doctors' appointments, so we could not avoid the car.

    Then there was the problem of eating. I was still pumping breast milk for Jaclyn, and she was drinking it from bottles. The doctors had determined how many ounces of breast milk she needed per day. She wasn't consuming nearly as much milk as they wanted her to have, so her growth and weight gain were a struggle. Drinking from bottles was still very difficult for her. Jaclyn would drink a little and then fall asleep. Her heart was working so hard that her body was burning more calories than she was taking in. I was provided with many tricks to try to keep her awake so she could eat; none worked. I flicked her foot. I undressed her in hopes that being cold would keep her awake. I put water on her face. Feeding Jaclyn was becoming more and more stressful.

Over and over again we were reminded of the importance of Jaclyn's growth. If she didn't eat, she wouldn't grow. If she didn't grow, her arteries wouldn't grow. If her arteries didn't grow, there was little that could be done for her. The burden of Jaclyn's eating fell squarely on my shoulders.

During the whole eating ordeal, we were told that, if need be, we could resort to a feeding tube. Alan and I fought this notion. A gastro-tube, inserted into the abdominal wall, requires surgery. We were told these tubes occasionally came out, necessitating additional surgeries to replace them. The idea of a nasal-gastric tube was presented to us as well. This tube would be placed down the nose and throat and into the stomach so milk could be syringed into the tube at feeding time. We did not like this option either, so we continued to endure stressful feedings in order to avoid the need for a feeding tube.

I continued to use the pump many times every day for five months. Because Jaclyn wasn't eating as much as I was pumping, I had enough frozen breast milk to last for nine months.

Over the years, that burden of getting calories into Jaclyn's body has still primarily been mine. By September, at age four months, eating was still a nightmare. I hated the pressure of trying to get Jaclyn to consume calories. I had a ritual of singing her a made-up song, bouncing her in my arms, and walking in circles through my house while I gave her a bottle. I sang the same ridiculous song, over and over and over. I had convinced myself that she drank more when we adhered to this pattern. In retrospect, I don't know what I was thinking. But in those moments of utter craziness, I believe that people tell themselves anything, no matter how illogical, in order to get through a stressful time.

Sometimes I would get so anxious at bottle time that I would call relatives to come over and feed Jaclyn, just so I wouldn't have to do it. I got to the point where pumping milk and spending increasingly long amounts of time trying to feed her milk took up the bulk of my days.

The saving grace during those chaotic, difficult moments was my beautiful, happy baby. Despite it all, Jaclyn was easy-going. She was interested in my face, my voice, my words, my songs. I couldn't get enough of her. I believe her attitude, even as a baby, made it less stressful when caring for her.

In September, Jaclyn contracted a respiratory infection, which made it nearly impossible for her to eat and breathe at the same time. Obviously, breathing was the priority. We opted for the non-surgical feeding tube, the nasal-gastric kind. Reluctantly, we went back to the hospital for its insertion. I watched the nurse put the tube down Jaclyn's nose and heard my daughter choke on it as she swallowed. The nurse continued feeding the tube into Jaclyn's nose so it would go all the way to her stomach. When Jaclyn screamed, I cried. Never in my wildest dreams did I realize I would have to learn how to insert the tube, nor that I would have to change it regularly.

We could not leave the hospital until both Alan and I learned how to insert the nasal-gastric (NG) tube, which meant practicing on Jaclyn. The nurse went over the steps, one at a time. First, we had to measure the distance from Jaclyn's nose to her ear, which represented the length to the back of her throat. Then we measured from her ear down her chest, to about an inch below her sternum. This was how far we had to insert the tube so it would go in her nose, down her throat, and into her stomach. Next we prepared special orange tape which secured the tube to Jaclyn's nose. On the short end of the rectangular piece of tape we had cut, we made a ¾ inch slit, leaving the rest of the tape intact. After putting petroleum jelly on the end of the tube, we were ready to insert it.

We lay Jaclyn down on a table and had to tilt her head backward in order to make it easier for her to swallow the tube. As we would begin to put the tube into one nostril, we would encounter resistance when the tube reached her throat. We were taught to push through this resistance, often causing a brief choke or gag reflex as she swallowed the tube. We continued fishing in the tube, until coming to the spot measured earlier. This was all being done on an often screaming and squirming child. Jaclyn would shriek and turn red, she'd twist her head quickly back and forth so we couldn't get the tube in, she'd kick and try to roll off the table, and she'd gag and occasionally vomit. It was torture to do this to Jaclyn and a truly horrid experience for us.

The next step was taping the tube. The uncut end of the orange tape needed to be placed on the tip of the nose, with the slits pointing down toward the lip. One slit was wrapped a number of times, clockwise, around the tube. The other slit was wrapped counter-clockwise. One end of the tube was now in the stomach. The other end came out of Jaclyn's nose, and we were taught to drape it to her ear and secure it with a little piece of paper tape. We rolled the remaining inches of tube into a loose circle and taped it to the back of Jaclyn's clothes.

The final step was to check the placement of the tube to be sure it was in her stomach. We learned to use a stethoscope and to push a puff of air through a syringe into the tube. With the stethoscope placed on Jaclyn's stomach, we were able to hear a 'whiff' as the air went in. If we didn't hear this sound, the tube was placed improperly and would need to be removed and re-inserted.

It was time to practice putting the tube in ourselves. Alan went first, mostly because I refused. He did it correctly the first time while I stood against the wall, watching in horror. I told the nurse that I would not need to learn this, as it was clear my husband would be able to insert it. I was informed that, when Alan was not home, Jaclyn could accidentally pull out the tube, that it could become clogged and therefore unusable, and that it would need to be replaced monthly with a new tube. I asked if I could bring Jaclyn to the hospital if the tube came out and have nurses reinsert it, but that request was rejected. As my hands shook, and the feeling of hopelessness coarsed through my veins, I inserted the tube. Jaclyn choked. Jaclyn cried. Tears filled my eyes. When it was in correctly, I got hysterical for having had to perform an act this horrific on my child. Then we went home.

The idea behind the feeding tube was that once the respiratory infection was over, Jaclyn would be better able to eat on her own. Plus, the extra calories could only help. However, that's not what happened. Shortly after getting the tube, she began choking when we gave her a pacifier. She was losing the ability to suck. The gastroenterologist, the doctor who had initiated the NG-tube, felt there was nothing we could do at this time. In his words, "breathing was still of primary importance, as feeding was being taken care of."

It was my fault the first time Jaclyn's NG-tube came out. I had inadvertently rolled her onto the tube while changing her diaper, and it slipped right out of her nose. I was petrified at the prospect of having to put the tube back in myself. I was home with her alone. I thought about begging Alan to come home from work to do it but then felt guilty for not being able to take care of my own child. I didn't want Jaclyn to miss a feeding, so I talked myself into it and decided it was time to be in control.

I lay Jaclyn on the changing table and got my supplies ready. It took me more than one try to insert the tube. Each time I tried to get the tube past the back of her throat, she cried and squirmed. She lifted her legs to try to push me away. I couldn't do it. I started to panic, which only made it worse. The more she cried, the more upset I became. Shaking, I somehow got the damn tube in all the way. I was relieved, but at the same time, I was angry that I had to do that to her. Jaclyn did not deserve this. The unfairness of everything was overwhelming.

So the feeding tube stayed. It was part of our lives from the time Jaclyn was four months old to the age of 2 ½ years! It is one of the things I have simply put out of my mind. Thinking back on it now just seems surreal. I can't believe she had a feeding tube that long, and I can't believe we made it through. Other than Alan and I, the only other person who learned how to put in Jaclyn's NG-tube was my mom. Though reluctant and angry about having to do this to her grandchild, she did it for my husband and for me. She did it so we could leave Jaclyn with her and go out for some couple time.

Unfortunately, with the feeding tube came other issues. First there was the staring. I had this amazingly beautiful child, with huge brownish/hazel eyes, a full head of thick dark brown hair, long eyelashes, perfectly shaped eyebrows, a teeny nose, and a little rosebud mouth. But nobody saw that when I took her out. They saw orange tape on the tip of her nose and a tube sticking out of it. For many months I didn't take Jaclyn out often, except to visit relatives. After awhile I got tired of being indoors, and we'd go walking around the neighborhood. This wasn't so bad. In the winter we started going for walks inside the mall. Most of the time people would just stare, and we would go on our way. Other times children, and occasionally adults, would ask about the tube. I would explain that it was a feeding tube, and people would say "aw" and walk away. Sometimes we could feel people's eyes following us. Once a woman literally walked into a beam in the mall because she was more focused on Jaclyn's nose than where she was going. This irritated me, although I somewhat understood. What annoyed me the most were the insensitive parents who would shoo their children away from our stroller or say "there must be something wrong with her."

With the feeding tube also came reflux. Feeding Jaclyn now meant opening the end of the tube, which was taped to her clothes, and syringing breast milk (and later, formula) into the tube. We knew exactly how much she was supposed to have each day, and we divided it among feedings. However, Jaclyn started to experience reflux. What I'd put in, she'd spit up. And not little episodes of spitting up; we were living with projectile vomiting! I tried feeding her less milk, more often, but that didn't work. I tried different formulas, to no avail. I fed her more slowly, which only made the feedings take up more of the day, with no success. After several visits to different gastroenterologists, she was put on two reflux medications, bringing the total number of medicines each day to five. These did not work either.

Now that Jaclyn was bigger, she could sit better in the car seat so I didn't need a travel companion all the time. But the reflux made driving interesting. Jaclyn was still facing backwards in her car seat. I became quite adept at reaching my arm back to her and holding a cloth for her to spit up in, while I was driving.

Next came the arrival of our third piece of medical equipment: a Kangaroo pump. During the day, Jaclyn couldn't take in all the formula I was syringing into her because she would throw it up. The doctors decided that half of her calories could be pumped into her NG-tube while she slept at night. Now, in addition to oximeter alarm bells, we had the added bonus of beeping noises when the Kangaroo pump erred, emptied, or clogged during the night.

Lessons Jaclyn Taught Me.

One's tolerance level is often higher than one thinks. The first few times I had to insert the NG-tube, both Jaclyn and I became hysterical. As she got older, she got more used to the tube and eventually learned to lay still for its insertion. Not only did this make it easier on her, but on me as well. We got through it because we had no choice. But it became less of an ordeal because she was able to tolerate it, and therefore so was I. What used to be a horrible and dreaded experience eventually became manageable. This was true for many of the medical issues that were thrown our way as Jaclyn got older.

You Know It's a Problem When...

Having your child in the hospital is never fun. Being admitted into ICU and having nurses and medical residents greet you by name because they have seen you so often is even worse. Jaclyn was sick a lot during her first year. She was born in May, diagnosed in early June, had her first surgery later in June, and by fall she had experienced numerous respiratory infections, pneumonia, and respiratory syncytial virus (RSV). She was admitted to the hospital many times. The nurses began to include Alan and me in their dinner plans. If they were going to order food to be delivered to the hospital, they offered to add our order to theirs. After all, we were on "The Unit" (ICU) around the clock. We were becoming regulars on the floor of the pediatric ICU.

When new residents and interns came through the unit for rounds, they were always fascinated with Jaclyn. They would spend longer than normal amounts of time listening to her heart with their stethoscopes, simply because her various murmurs were intriguing. I detested the fact that my child was a test case for them.

When Jaclyn was hospitalized, I would call my mother who lived out of state. I felt guilty because I knew she would fly back and help me—and she did just that. As soon as Jaclyn would recover, my mom would head back to California, awaiting the next illness. I felt terrible about this; however, my mom would never have had it any other way.

The reality of more hospitalizations, more procedures, and

more surgeries was always on my mind. The risks that Jaclyn would have to be exposed to were ever-present. I got to a point where I would be driving in my car, and if I passed a cemetery, I would become anxious. I would get uncomfortable and fidgety in my seat. It was completely irrational. The doctors had already told us that Jaclyn's anatomy made cardiac repairs 'doable.' But somehow, I still had that surgeon's words in my head—that I could go home without my baby. It was many years before I could drive by a cemetery and not have to turn away to distract myself.

Trying To Be "Normal"

Between the first and second surgeries, we learned more about pulmonary atresia and Jaclyn's other heart anomalies. Having a child with a chronic condition often took over the majority of my days. While my husband was back into his regular work schedule and my mother had gone home, my days were focused solely on Jaclyn. I took an indefinite leave of absence from my postdoctoral fellowship. My days were filled with Jaclyn—caring for her, playing with her, taking her to and from appointments, feeding her, and being with her.

From the time she awoke in the morning to the time she went to bed at night, I was constantly on vigil. I knew what time it was at any given moment of each and every day. This was critical. I had to know when it was time for her morning doses of medications. I had to wait at least one hour before administering her second set of morning medications because they could not be taken together. I was still tube-feeding her on a schedule, and she was refluxing after meals. It was still critical to be sure a good amount of calories stayed in her body for growth, even if that meant feeding her additional amounts right after she refluxed. If I had to run errands, they had to be timed precisely so as not to interfere with eating or refluxing. This meant I could take Jaclyn with me to the grocery store, or to the doctor, or wherever, during select hours of the morning. We had to be back at set times too.

Afternoons weren't much different. Jaclyn would be tube fed

again around lunch time. Her afternoon nap sometimes eased the reflux. The less movement she had post-feedings, the better it seemed to be. Again, this required timing on my part. If I took her out, it had to be after lunch and nap, which meant late afternoon. She needed mid-afternoon medications, and these needed to be refrigerated. So going out in the afternoons meant I had to be sure to bring an ice pack and syringes of medications with me. There were simply not enough hours in the day in which to spread her medications if I were to accidentally miss a dose.

Meanwhile, despite my focus on Jaclyn's medical needs, now that she was almost six months old, she required more stimulation. This was the part I loved, and this is where she thrived. Jaclyn couldn't move very well, so she spent a good portion of her days lying on her back. She hated to be on her stomach, despite encouragement to do so from doctors. She couldn't roll over and crawling was not going to be in our future. One day I bought Jaclyn a helium-filled balloon. While lying on her back, she became fascinated tugging on the balloon's ribbon and watching the balloon move closer, then farther, then closer again. Balloons became part of our play from that point on.

There we were at home, Jaclyn recovering from her first surgery when she was six weeks old and a second surgery date not yet scheduled. During the next weeks and months, Jaclyn and I got busy being normal. Thus began our indulgence in books. To read to her, I would sometimes prop her between my legs. Other times I would lay her on her back, on a mat on the floor. I'd then lie on my back beside her, holding a book over our heads to read. Since my mother collects children's books, we were never lacking for new reading material. Jaclyn kicked her legs in response to pictures, she reached her arms up toward the books, she squealed as I read, and she seemed fascinated by the voices I made and the pictures she saw. This was a favorite activity, and we engaged in it all the time. As more weeks and months passed, Jaclyn began to reach out to books as if to turn the pages. She shrieked with delight, only encouraging me, or my husband, or aunts, cousins, grandparents and great grandparents to read to her more and more.

When my mom was in California, she used to read Dr. Seuss' *Yertle the Turtle* to Jaclyn over the telephone. This book and *The Three Little Pigs* were among Jaclyn's favorites—we read them over and over again.

We also spent our days listening to music. We listened to children's tapes, with silly lyrics and rhymes, and they made Jaclyn take notice. She was only a few months old, but it was obvious that she wanted more. We sang, we laughed, she bopped along, and we healed.

Trying to be "normal" also meant going for long walks, or sitting her on the patio and watching the leaves blow. Relatives would often come over to visit. We tried to visit great grandmothers or my aunt as often as we could, but it was difficult with the feeding and refluxing schedule we were on. A lot of the time, Jaclyn and I were alone together during the day. At some point she noticed television. I remember watching the Olympics' opening ceremony in August, 1996, and seeing Jaclyn's eyes transfixed by the screen. There were sparkling lights, fireworks, and flags. She couldn't get enough.

I mentioned to Alan that Jaclyn noticed television for the first time, only to have him inform me she had been watching David Letterman at night with him for weeks. Our routine was that I went to bed around 9:00 or 10:00 pm. Alan stayed up late to work, with Jaclyn on his lap or over his shoulder while at his computer. Sometimes they'd watch late-night television together, unbeknownst to me. Maybe Jaclyn's love for staying up late began with her dad and David Letterman.

When Jaclyn was only a few months old, we also began to do puzzles. At first we worked on simple eight-piece puzzles with big knobs on each piece. I'd sit Jaclyn on my lap or in between my legs and dump out the pieces. Then I would hold her hand on a knob, with my hand over it, and we would try to put the pieces into each hole. "Does this fit?" I'd ask. "No." "Does it go here?" "No." "Here?" "Yes!" She'd laugh when it fit. Of course she was young to be doing puzzles, but it was something to do and a new challenge to be met. Who's to say that her ability to master 100-piece puzzles by age four was not attributable to her early start?

Tucked away in a drawer, I had been keeping the names and phone numbers of two families whose children had cardiac anomalies similar to Jaclyn's. The surgeon's assistant had given me the names as a kind of support. For months I had been too scared to call these people to ask what they had been through. Knowing the second surgery was coming was the motivation I needed to find out what this experience had been like for others. One day I picked one of the names and dialed the number. A woman answered the phone, and I explained that my daughter had recently undergone surgery similar to her child's cardiac repair. She didn't mind talking to me. I was terribly nervous but listened to her story with a pounding in my chest.

The woman told me that she had twin girls. One was born healthy, and the other, Lindsey, had five cardiac anomalies. Jaclyn had four; only one matched the type that Lindsey had. Knowing that our cases weren't identical was somehow comforting. After we rattled off the medical terminology for our respective children's difficulties, she began to speak more bluntly than I was prepared to hear. She told me that together, she and her husband had accepted "that G-d might take Lindsey" from them. Moreover, she said that "this was okay because it meant G-d must have had a plan." For a few moments I held that phone to my ear in complete silence. Not only didn't I agree with her, but I was angered by her opinion. While her spiritual views somehow comforted her, I was trembling at the notion that it would be all right to lose a child. I could not get off the telephone fast enough! I came up with an excuse to hang up. I never called the second family.

Days before Halloween, Jaclyn learned to sit up. She was almost six months old. She could not get to a sitting position by herself, but once we sat her up, she could balance and remain sitting. It was a very exciting milestone. She was not able to roll over because the first surgery cut through muscles on her left side. So sitting up was a big deal to us. She wore a pumpkin costume that first Halloween, and we proudly showed off her sitting-by-herself skill to anybody who would watch. We probably made a bigger deal out of Halloween than most first-time parents, but the next surgery was coming up soon. We learned to relish what precious "normal" moments we could.

Lessons Jaclyn Taught Me.

There are many things one can do, even when there are many things one cannot do. Don't dwell on the "cannots"; look hard to find the "cans."

Second Surgery is Scheduled

By November, 1996, Jaclyn was six months old and ready to undergo the second unifocalization of arteries, this time on the right side. Alan and I got as ready as we could, only to have Jaclyn contract pneumonia the week before the planned date. Surgery had to be rescheduled, the anticipation began again, and we waited six more weeks for her lungs to recover. Then she had the second unifocalization.

It was during this surgery that my ability to be nonjudgmental flew out the window. I remember sitting in the lobby of the hospital with various relatives during the actual surgery. For much of the time, we sat in silence. After a few hours of mindless chatter about the weather, sports, etc., people started to read books and magazines to help pass the time.

At some point, conversation turned to vacations. I remember sitting and listening to a family member's description of a recent wonderful trip. This seemed terribly insensitive to me as my daughter lay on an operating table with her body cut open. I realized people were only trying to pass the time, but this was a blunt reminder to me that very few people had any inkling about what our life was like. Vacations were far from our minds! Did I expect people to sulk the whole time Jaclyn was in surgery? At some level, I did expect others to be somewhat reserved while my daughter lay on an operating table. I didn't feel it was appropriate to sit in the waiting room laughing and sharing funny stories. Jaclyn wasn't having a good time, so why should we?

Rationally I know this thinking is selfish and ridiculous. After all, people deal with stress differently. I may sit quietly, while others talk to break the silence. Some people tell stories or even attempt humor. No one way to act in a hospital is correct, of course. While I know this intuitively to be true, I sometimes have to tune others out while I sit in that surgical waiting room—waiting and waiting, talking to G-d in my mind, sending Jaclyn messages to "stay strong." Listening to humorous stories or hearing others' exciting news just irritates me. I learned to deal with it, but it was never easy.

The second surgery introduced us to fluid retention. Jaclyn began retaining fluids a few days after the surgery. Her heart was having difficulty pumping efficiently, and subsequently her body couldn't rid itself of fluids. Her face puffed, her stomach distended; she didn't look like herself. Diuretics were administered then, and Jaclyn has remained on those diuretics ever since.

Although we had already been through one surgery, I still remember the queasy feeling I had the first time I saw the new incision. My daughter's soft, smooth skin had now been cut into again. The outcome was the same as the first surgery, but now on the right side—an incision about three inches under the right arm pit, a chest tube two inches below, a ventilator, and various IVs. She needed oxygen again at home for weeks after the surgery to allow her lungs time to heal. It was hard to fit an oxygen cannula in her tiny, little nose, in addition to her NG-feeding tube.

However, when this surgery was over, we knew we had a longer hiatus before the next one. It was a relief to bring Jaclyn home. We had been in the hospital for ten days this time.

Therapies Begin

After Jaclyn recovered from the second surgery, I became fanatical about beginning to address other problems we were facing. Jaclyn was seven months old, and the list of areas to conquer was staggering to me: she was not very mobile, rolling and crawling were not occurring, she couldn't eat, she had a feeding tube, and she never put toys in her mouth as other children did because they caused her to choke or gag. With encouragement from doctors, we began physical and occupational therapy. I had to fight to have speech therapy added to the mix, as a speech therapist is the person who could teach Jaclyn how to coordinate sucking, swallowing and breathing. I was desperate to address the eating problem that the gastroenterologist labeled as "the least of my worries." This was a doctor who had given my daughter a feeding tube, and then, when I asked him at follow-up how to get her off it, he told me that it was "not his problem!"

At first I brought Jaclyn to the hospital's therapy programs. Physical therapy was very hard for her. The therapist tried to teach her to crawl, or at least to move a knee and arm in an attempt to mimic crawling. But the muscles under Jaclyn's arms had been cut into during the first and second surgeries, making it difficult and perhaps painful for her to bear weight on them. This seemed to become less painful for Jaclyn as the months went on, but it was slow-go all the way. She never did crawl, though she was eventually able to scoot backwards on her butt. Very adaptive.

Speech therapy, on the other hand, was traumatic from the first day. The first therapist bounced Jaclyn on an oversized ball while rubbing Cheetos in her mouth. She did this for twenty minutes at a time, while my daughter choked, gagged, spit up, cried, and turned blue. She was trying to desensitize Jaclyn to having something in her mouth. The bouncing ball was supposed to help Jaclyn get comfortable being off-balance. My daughter's muscles had been very tight. She was sitting unassisted, but she could not get to that position by herself. She also could not pick herself up if she fell. The only form of movement she had was scooting on her behind. Consequently, she was very stiff and always perfectly upright. I didn't know whether this therapy made sense or not, but I went along with it for awhile. At less than a year old, Jaclyn started to wail as we approached the hospital parking lot for our scheduled therapy appointment. I think she wanted me to know how much she hated the speech therapy treatment.

I was on my own to find alternative therapists. Doctors gave me recommendations, but nobody had experience with a one year old who didn't know how to eat, couldn't crawl, roll, or move. I finally found a new speech therapist who became a savior. The first day we met this woman, she gave Jaclyn Colorforms to play with. After this distraction, she put a bubble blower, dipped in lemon juice, to Jaclyn's lips. Jaclyn didn't spit it out, gag or even throw it. Instead, she played with it on her lips, and when the woman guided it into her mouth, Jaclyn let her. This was the first time my child had put anything to her mouth since losing the ability to suck at about age five months. The therapist explained to me that plain tastes wouldn't excite or get Jaclyn's attention. It was the extreme flavors we would need to use to get her interested in food. Plus, a bubble blower was a textured item. It had ridges all around it, which could tingle the lips and tongue. This new experience intrigued Jaclyn.

First we saw the speech therapist weekly. Then we started to go twice a week, and for awhile she saw Jaclyn three times each week. As long as I was making the long drive to this woman's office, I eventually transferred Jaclyn's physical therapy to a therapist in that practice too. Just shy of turning one year old, Jaclyn could walk around furniture. At thirteen months she was taking steps unassisted. She still couldn't get to a standing position by herself, because that required using her arms to push her up, but she was definitely making progress.

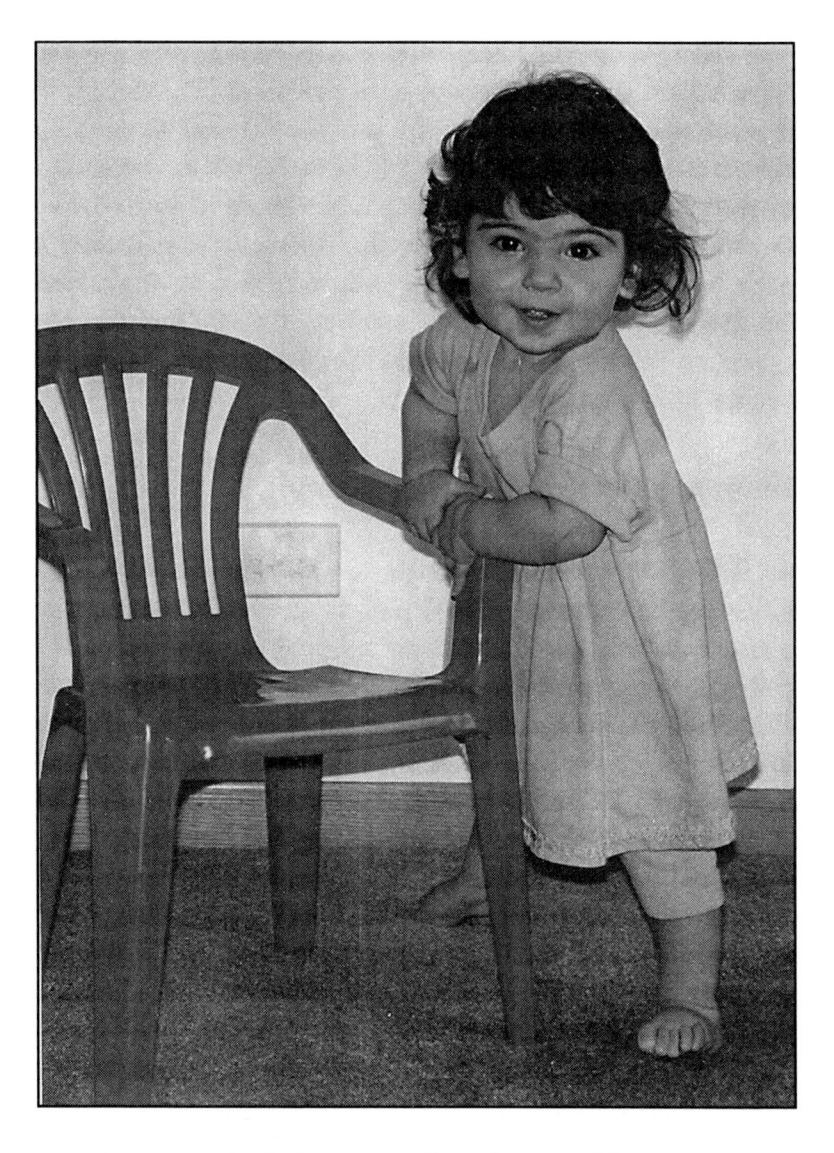

At 13 months, Jaclyn was walking but not able to get to a standing position by herself.

I continued to take Jaclyn to see this speech and physical therapist for years. It was there that she learned to stand up by herself. It was there that pickle juice, bubble soap, lemons, and pixie stick candies helped awaken my daughter to the wonders of taste. It took two years before she could actually eat, but this was where we met the woman who laid the groundwork for eating to later occur. It was there that Jaclyn rocked on a rocking horse alone and wasn't bothered about being off-balance. It was there that she mastered stair-climbing, though leading with the same leg each time instead of alternating them. Jaclyn came to love these therapists, as did I. They taught my daughter to do things other parents take for granted. To me, these therapists were life-savers!

Lessons Jaclyn Taught Me.

Even babies and toddlers have opinions that matter. Jaclyn clearly despised the first attempts at both physical therapy and occupational therapy. Not only did she become agitated as we'd approach the building for these appointments, but she'd also try to resist and refuse the treatments as her age, size and strength permitted. As her mother, I thought my job was to schedule appointments with recommended therapists, take Jaclyn to them, and assume these specialists knew best. Initially I didn't consider questioning their methods. But my one-year old daughter was trying to tell me, with her behavior, that these treatments were not acceptable. Once I caught on, I found other therapists who used alternative approaches, and Jaclyn began to progress. I learned the importance of taking cues from Jaclyn and really listening to her. She knew what felt comfortable for her own body. Of course, I couldn't oblige her every demand, as no parent can or should, but her opinion did deserve to be heard and attended to, when possible. This lesson served us well as other medical problems arose.

Just Being a Kid

In addition to the medical needs, Jaclyn was still a curious one-year old. She would walk around the house, often attached to the Kangaroo feeding pump which was hung on a portable IV pole with wheels. Sometimes I resorted to using the feeding pump, rather than syringing milk into her tube, because it allowed me a few free moments. However, I would have to keep close watch on Jaclyn as she moved, so she wouldn't walk too far from the pole, either pulling out the connector and spraying milk all over the house, or toppling the IV pole onto herself. I often just followed behind her, pushing the pole so she could finish an NG-tube feeding. Visitors used to question why I didn't put Jaclyn in a high chair while the pump was on. But feeding took so long, and I saw how excited she was to move freely about the house after being relatively immobile for so long. So I let her enjoy her new-found freedom as often as I could.

By now, we had added lots of new experiences to our life, and Jaclyn was happy to play with anyone who came over to visit. We played house, kitchen, dollhouse, puppets, restaurant, and grocery store. She loved to pick out plastic play food to buy, put it in a shopping cart, pay for it with paper money in a toy cash register, and load it into the Cozy Coupe car that she "drove" home. We finger-painted and began delving into crafts of all kinds. We also played dress-up with my mom's fancy jewelry. Jaclyn couldn't get enough of wearing clip-on earrings and bunches of necklaces and bracelets at the same time. She didn't like the costume (fake) stuff—just the real jewelry.

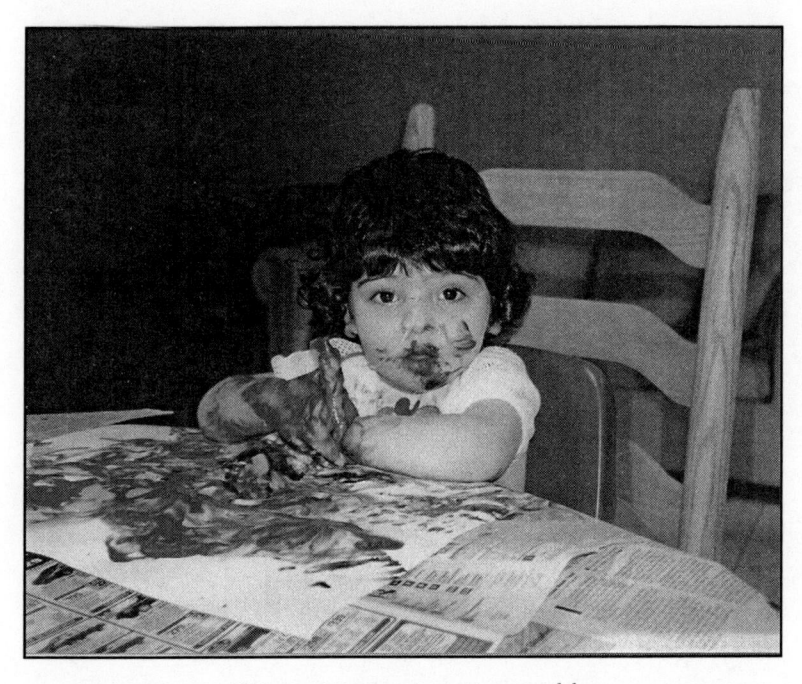

Fingerpainting at one year old.

Although Jaclyn understood everything, sounds and speech were slow to come for her. I worried that the feeding tube would affect her speech, but the speech therapist working with us on eating was also teaching me how to work with Jaclyn on sounds. I would sit Jaclyn on the bathroom vanity, standing behind to hold her, and we would look into the mirror together to make silly faces and to produce sounds.

We also sang a lot—a huge repertoire of children's songs I had memorized. Jaclyn would bounce, bending her knees and straightening them to the beat. I also tried some of the eating tactics at home, but Jaclyn wanted nothing to do with them. She let the therapist fiddle with her mouth during appointments, but home was strictly for fun.

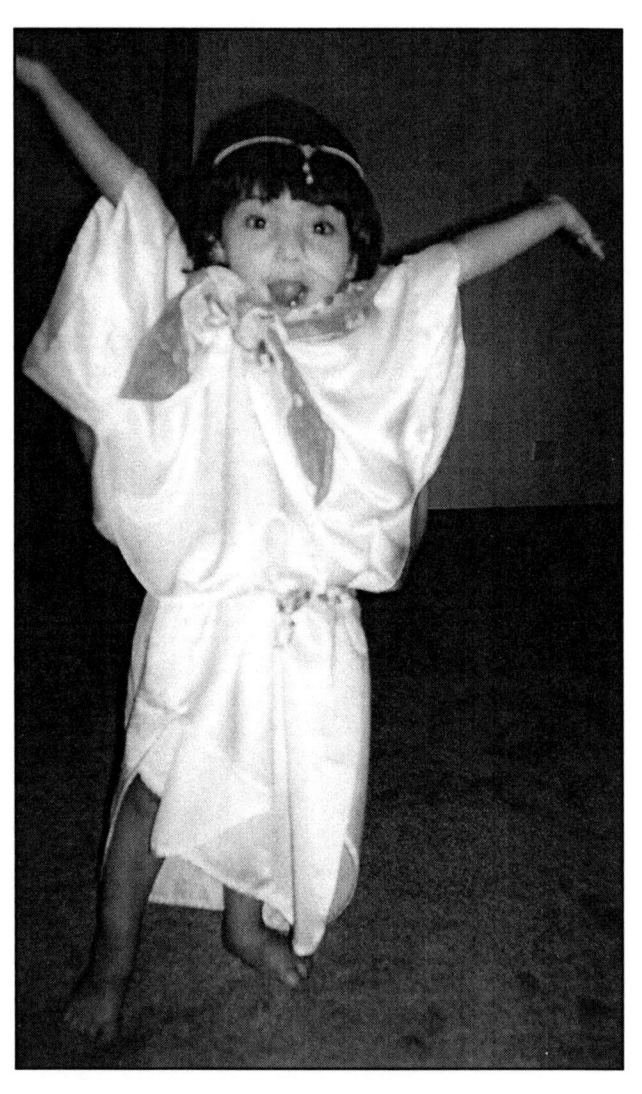

She loved to dress up and ham it up for the camera. Age 2.

Third Surgery: The Big One

At 18 months of age, Jaclyn would undergo her first open-heart surgery. The surgeon's explanation of what would be attempted was terrifying to me. It was before this big surgery that I began a ritual I secretly maintained for years. Many days before a hospitalization, while Jaclyn was asleep, I would sit on her bed, rubbing her back, smoothing her hair, and I would talk to her. I would tell her that I knew she was strong, that she could come through whatever the next procedure or surgery was, and that she would be okay.

Then, I would talk to G-d. I am not a very religious or spiritual person at all. In fact, since Jaclyn's diagnosis I found myself not really happy with G-d for making my daughter go through all that she had. So talking to G-d was definitely a significant step for me. I would ask G-d to please look after Jaclyn during the next procedure or surgery and to look after the surgeon too. I would pray that my daughter would be all right when it was over. And then I would add, "And, please, dear G-d, let her come through this with no disabling disabilities." I wanted assurances that no complications would occur during or after surgery. So I asked, over and over again, for "no disabling disabilities"—this was the phrase I came up with and used for every surgery and procedure.

There are always anesthesia risks associated with surgery. It was explained to us that air could get into a catheter and go to the patient's brain. My child's personality was shining through. She was sweet, she was smart, and I wanted to be sure we did everything we could to nurture and care for those abilities. "No disabling disabilities"—these are words I uttered, day after day, night after night, before any and all procedures or surgeries. While we sat in the surgical family waiting room when she was actually in surgery, I repeated these words over and over in my mind. When things were so out of my control, this was one small thing I could do.

When a mother tells others that her daughter is going to have open-heart surgery, people think they know what that means. I have learned that many people believe open-heart surgery is so common today that the patient is home in a matter of days and back to their old selves in no time! For some people, heart surgery and recovery is that kind of miracle. But that has never happened for Jaclyn. People do not understand the complexity of Jaclyn's surgeries, and sometimes their comments end up minimizing my fear. I realize people don't know Jaclyn's anatomy, how much "repair" work really needs to be done, how risky it is, or how miraculous the technology is to accomplish it all. I don't fault people for their lack of understanding. But as absurd as it sounds, "she'll be fine" offers no relief to me, even from well-meaning people.

By the time Jaclyn was ready for this third surgery, our favorite surgeon had his own pediatric surgical heart unit (PSHU) at his hospital. We took Jaclyn to his hospital and never had contact with the other surgeon again. However, by going there we gave up the convenience of being close to home. Despite now travelling forty-four miles one way from our home to this new hospital, we made the decision to have this big surgery completed on the surgeon's "home turf" because it seemed better for Jaclyn.

Once we were on the PSHU unit, we knew we had made the right choice. All the nurses on the unit were cardiac nurses, and we learned quickly how much of a difference this makes. In contrast, in the hospital where Jaclyn's first two surgeries were performed, she would recover in a regular pediatric ICU. There, nurses often panicked when Jaclyn's oxygen saturations dropped. On the new unit, there were no children with pneumonia or RSV or other regular ICU diagnoses. Instead, Jaclyn was on a unit with only cardiac kids who, as we learned, present their own unique challenges. Nurses equipped for just that specialty made an amazing difference.

There have always been jitters and upset stomachs the days

before surgery. When Jaclyn was a toddler, we used to tell her about surgeries or procedures two or three days in advance. That way, we could talk about it, give her time to think about it, and also give her a chance to formulate questions if she needed to. This wasn't much of an issue when she was under three, but after that age, she did start to remember hospitalizations and did have questions. Mostly, she asked if she would need an IV because she hated that the most. We reminded her that she would be sleeping while the doctor worked "to fix her heart." She wanted to be sure we'd be there when she awoke. When she was younger, she also wanted to make sure we remembered to pack her favorite blanket and stuffed animals. Those were her questions and concerns. As she got older, the litany of questions encompassed weeks instead of days. Jaclyn processed, asked, examined diagrams of her heart versus a "normal" heart, and tried to understand, from our explanations, what would really be happening.

Because this was open-heart surgery, it was riskier than previous surgeries, so the protocol was a bit different beforehand. This time, we were asked to quarantine Jaclyn and ourselves for the week leading up to the surgery. If Jaclyn developed so much as a drippy nose any time during the preceding ten days, the surgery would be cancelled and not take place for at least two weeks, or until she was completely recovered.

This request to stay home made sense logically, but psychologically it was taxing on us. Alan tried to work at home as often as possible, but there were days when he had to go to his office. Upon returning home at the end of the day, I would be crazed at the thought of the germs he had come into contact with at work. When he walked in the door, he would immediately wash his hands and change clothes before he could even kiss Jaclyn or me hello. Relatives dropped groceries off at our door and waved to Jaclyn and me, two caged beings stuck in a house. Halloween fell during that quarantine week. Jaclyn loved watching Sherri Lewis and Lambchop videos. My mom made a fuzzy Lambchop costume. However, other than my husband and me, nobody actually saw Jaclyn in the costume up close. Instead, we sat in the window and waved, as my mom, grandmother, and aunt drove by the house to see her in her costume and to blow her kisses through the window.

We survived the quarantine, and Jaclyn was healthy. However, life was still out of our control. The day before the surgery was to take place, we got a call from the surgeon's liaison informing us that surgery had to be rescheduled. The donated pulmonary artery and valve to be used in Jaclyn's heart were not available. We had built up for this day, even quarantined ourselves, only to have to reschedule and anticipate a new surgery date. It was maddening, but there was nothing we could do about it.

After three weeks of waiting, surgery day finally arrived. This surgery was called a Rastelli. It involved taking the two sets of arteries that had previously been unifocalized under Jaclyn's arms and connecting them to a donated pulmonary artery and pulmonary valve to her heart, since she was born without these. Sitting in the waiting room during the actual surgery was a real test of nerves. Again, various family members were there with us. It was a very long day. After nearly eight hours, we went to see Jaclyn and were shocked at her appearance. She was lying on her back, with the standard IVs, catheters, and ventilator that she would need to be on for several days while she began to recover. She was puffed up from being on the heart/lung machine too.

Our families went out to dinner that first night. It was a break from the hospital after a terribly long day and also a respite before the long journey of recovery still yet to come. Eating that first night, not even aware of how famished we were, we had no idea what a difficult recovery lay ahead for her or for us. We were soon to find out.

For the first two surgeries, Jaclyn came off the ventilator rather quickly—usually the next morning. But this time she needed to be on the ventilator much longer, which was difficult because she was older and more aware of things. The ventilator was horrendous because the tube down her throat meant she couldn't talk or even make a sound. The hardest part of those hospital days for me was watching her fight that machine. In order to come off a ventilator, one's body has to be awake enough to take over the job of breathing. Jaclyn was waking up and struggling to pull the tube out of her throat. Nurses put restraints on her arms. This seemed merciless to me.

Also, because she was more awake and more aware, Jaclyn began to move around in the bed. Thrashing in the hospital bed made the tube in her throat move around, causing her to gag and choke. The choking was problematic because she could aspirate. The nurse needed to calm her down. But it was almost impossible to explain to a 1 ½ year old that she would feel better if she stopped moving and crying. Jaclyn was sore, tired, and terribly frightened. When she would cry, no sound was emitted because the ventilator was down her throat. Tears of fear came out of Jaclyn's eyes. These moments were hardest for us to watch. We sat at her bedside, trying to sing to her, talk to her, and soothe her in order to get through this awful ventilator experience. If the doctors sedated her too much, we'd have to begin the weaning process again.

Once the ventilator experience was over, Jaclyn began retaining fluids. She was already on diuretics to help rid her body of excess fluids. This was familiar ground for us, as the same issue had occurred before. For a few days the doctors played with diuretic doses and types. Finally they found one that seemed to help. However, it was later determined that fluid was also accumulating around her heart. This was very dangerous and would need to be drained. It was a major set-back. A small tube had to be inserted into Jaclyn's chest, and the fluid was drained. This procedure sounded dreadful. We were very anxious as she underwent this additional procedure. But it took care of the problem, and recovery then continued.

For over three weeks Jaclyn stayed in ICU. Alan and I never left. We had simply moved in to her room and to the hospital's "Guest House" across the street. The Guest House was literally a house located across the parking lot from the hospital entrance. Families of children in the ICU or PSHU could stay there for $5/night. Each family had a bedroom of their own, with individual locks on the doors. All families shared the common rooms: bathrooms, kitchen and living room. We simply used the bedroom for a place to take turns sleeping each night (one of us always staying with Jaclyn), and the bathroom for showering each morning. While the house was convenient, we never spent any other time there, partly because it wasn't so clean, but also because we simply stayed with Jaclyn in her room all day and into the nights.

During that three week period, we developed a pattern. My mom would arrive at the hospital in the morning and stay until dinner time. Then she'd make the long drive home. Alan's parents and other relatives would often come on weekends and stay with us too. After Alan and I spent all day with Jaclyn in PSHU, he would walk me across the street to the Guest House, and I would go to sleep around 10:00 pm. He would return to Jaclyn's bedside. I would set an alarm for 3:00 or 4:00 am in order to relieve Alan. He would update me about how Jaclyn's night had gone so far—if there were any problems, if she had been awake and restless, or if she had been primarily sleeping. In the morning Alan would shower and return to the hospital. I would then go back to the Guest House to shower and dress. The first few nights after surgery we were both able to sleep in the Guest House because Jaclyn was sedated and not in danger of waking during the night and wondering where we were. After those first nights, our sleeplessness began. We just couldn't imagine coming home without our child. We both felt we wanted and needed to be with her at the hospital every day and night. So we stayed in the Guest House. For three weeks we stayed.

Thanksgiving came and went. Jaclyn was still in PSHU. My aunt and uncle were having holiday dinner at their house, and they wanted to cancel it because we couldn't come. Instead, they had an early dinner, and my mom brought Thanksgiving leftovers to us. While we appreciated her efforts, in all honesty sitting in the Guest House kitchen eating warmed-up turkey while my daughter was across the street in the hospital was a terribly depressing evening. It would be the first of many events and family get-togethers that we would miss, either due to Jaclyn's illness, quarantine periods, surgeries, or recoveries.

To pass three weeks of time in a little hospital room, Jaclyn listened to her favorite music and watched lots of videos. We read her many, many books. She was only 1 ½ years old, and there wasn't much else to do with her while she was stuck in an ICU bed with tubes and wires attached to her body. It was a brutal three weeks!

Finally, Jaclyn came home. Recovery was a long process, and her breastbone still needed to heal. We could not lift her under her arms for over three more weeks. We had to pick her up under her behind. Her heart and lungs needed to recover from the stress of the surgery and what strength she had built up in therapy was gone. But at least we were in our own house. Life would, once again, get back to "normal," although what was normal was changing slightly each time we would come home from a hospital stay. Now, "normal" included more medications, with more dosages throughout the day, and carrying Jaclyn everywhere so as not to let her fall and injure herself. Although she was sore, she was only 1 ½ and didn't understand that lying still would help her feel better faster. As a parent, it was difficult to try to stop her from getting around and not hovering over her. But hover I did. She wasn't out of my sight for weeks!

Revising the Life Plan

After Jaclyn's initial diagnosis at one month of age, I had taken an indefinite leave of absence from my postdoctoral fellowship. My advisors had been very accommodating to me during Jaclyn's surgeries and recoveries, but they eventually needed to know whether I planned to complete my two-year position or not. I was not able to commit to returning at any particular time, especially because more surgeries, more complicated ones with longer recovery times, were coming down the line. So, reluctantly, I gave up my fellowship.

This was a terribly depressing time for me. I kept replaying in my mind the first day that I had stepped onto campus to begin my postdoctoral fellowship. A bus had dropped me off, and I stood looking at the ivy-covered buildings of the University of Chicago. I stood in the center of what is called the Midway Plaisance and tears streamed down my cheeks. I was proud of the fact that I had made it to that point. I had gotten a Ph.D. from the top-rated program in my field. I had glowing recommendations from professors I admired. I had received a grant and also published more papers than other graduate students had. My work had been accepted at conferences for presentation. I had won awards. I was beginning a prestigious postdoctoral fellowship at a fabulous university. And also on that first day, I was excited at the prospect of being pregnant with my first child. My life was certainly everything I could have imagined. Giving up my fellowship was a sad—but necessary—step in my life.

When Jaclyn was just over two years of age, I received a phone call from a man offering me a job. I told him I was not looking for a position and asked how he got my name. Apparently he had read a journal article I had previously published, and he called the University of Chicago to track me down. When he found out I was no longer employed there, he asked for my contact information. They gave him my home phone number. He explained that my research was exactly what he had been looking for. He worked at the Rush Alzheimer's Disease Center in Chicago (RADC) and was in search of a researcher interested in family caregiving and Alzheimer's Disease. That description fit the person I used to be. Again I told him I was not looking for a job. He was persistent.

As a way to get this man off my back, I began to explain to him that my daughter had special medical needs and that I could not consider working full-time. He asked how many days I would prefer to work, part-time. I informed him that my daughter would require additional surgeries to repair her heart. He said I could have all the time off I would need during her surgery and recovery. He was willing to accommodate every obstacle I made to dissuade his pursuit of me. I felt as if this opportunity, which literally fell out of the sky and into my lap, was indeed worth a try.

In earnest, I began my search for someone to care for Jaclyn so I could go back to work part-time. Because she was still very susceptible to germs, a daycare center filled with many children was out of the question. I briefly considered hiring a nanny but didn't for a few reasons. First, if there was going to be a single person caring for my daughter, one-on-one, I wanted that person to be me. Second, if we were going to resort to some kind of daycare arrangement, I thought one-on-one care was too limited, as Jaclyn had been isolated from groups as a baby and toddler. I wasn't in denial about my child's health, but I did want her to have some interaction with other children. Our pediatrician also thought it would be beneficial for Jaclyn to be around small groups of children to start building up her immunities. I focused on finding a small home daycare setting.

I obtained a list of state-licensed home daycare providers in my area. The list had twenty-eight names on it. Many providers were not interested in taking children part-time; they only wanted kids who came five days a week. I crossed off those names. Other providers were already operating at full-capacity. The list began to narrow.

By looking at Jaclyn, no one could determine that she had any physical problems (except for the NG-tube). However, I was nervous about having to tell daycare providers about her medical history. I would certainly have to inform them that she would need medications during the day. That didn't worry me. I would also have to ascertain their protocol for sick children; for instance, would there be children with drippy noses in the daycare? The answer was "yes" to runny noses, but "no" to children with fevers. I learned that payment was still expected whenever your child was sick. I knew that Jaclyn would inevitably be sick a lot, and that, for her, a cold often caused a respiratory infection, which usually meant a fever. Our pediatrician had explained to us that Jaclyn's fevers were just her lungs' way of dealing with infections. She wasn't contagious; this was just how her lungs reacted. However, children with fevers were not welcome in home daycares. That meant many potential days of paying for day care but keeping Jaclyn at home. I realized I would simply have to take that chance if I was going to go back to work.

There was one hurdle, however, that was much more difficult to overcome in my search for a home daycare provider. Jaclyn was still NG-tube fed. She continued to have that damn feeding tube sticking out of her nose, taped to the back of her clothes. While she had no other disabilities requiring special attention from a provider, the feeding tube was a definite deal-breaker over and over again. When I'd gently broach the subject of a feeding tube, most providers had no idea what I was talking about. I'd then hold my breath as I explained that the provider would have to syringe Jaclyn's milk into a tube that went down her nose and throat to her stomach.

It would be an understatement to say that reactions to this request weren't positive! Some daycare providers flat-out said they had no time for children with special needs. A few asked for more details to clarify what I meant and then said they didn't think it would work out. Others expressed disgust and simply hung up on me. One woman offered to meet in order to see firsthand how the feeding tube worked. I took Jaclyn to her home, partly optimistic, only to have her flinch as she watched me feed my child. She wasn't interested in having Jaclyn in her daycare. I had exhausted every name on my list of providers.

For days, the reality of my situation brought me to tears. I felt sorry for myself. I felt sorry for Jaclyn too, because only one person even agreed to meet this bright, amazing, good-natured, happy, easy-going child. But she, too, wouldn't attempt the tube feedings. Instead, all people heard or saw was a sick child. I faced the prospect of never being able to work, because nobody was willing or able to give Jaclyn the care she required. My career dreams were slipping away, and there was nothing I could do about it. I was angry; angry at myself because I knew Jaclyn hadn't asked for this, angry at my husband because his career wasn't being stifled, and angry at the world in general.

A few days later, I got a phone call from a daycare provider. She had been on vacation and was just now returning my call. It seemed like a miracle was happening. Yes, she took part-time children. Yes, she had an opening. She didn't cut me off when I explained Jaclyn's feeding needs. Her own son had been born prematurely, and she was sensitive to special needs. She was willing to meet us.

When the day arrived for our visit, I prepared myself for another let-down. I took Jaclyn inside this woman's house. We went into the playroom. It was immaculate. Children sat on chairs at a small table working on puzzles and coloring. The woman bottle-fed an infant on her lap as we spoke. She was very gentle with the children. She asked some questions about Jaclyn's health. She was not alarmed by my responses. I explained that two medications would need to be administered, via tube, to Jaclyn during the day. I then described the mechanics of the feeding tube, waiting for a sign that she wasn't interested. She was not disgusted. She didn't foresee the tube as a hindrance. She was willing to give it a chance. I was speechless.

Jaclyn was now two years old, and I was able to go back to work three days a week. Jaclyn went to daycare two days each week, and my mom took care of her a third day. The daycare provider had a daughter who was the same age as Jaclyn, and they were buddies from day one. There were three other children in the daycare as well. This was exactly what Jaclyn needed. She was sick a lot, and it was a hassle when I had to explain that I couldn't come to work in order to care for her, but this was my child's first experience being around other children and doing things other children did. She thrived.

She's a Regular Kid After All

With three surgeries behind us, Jaclyn continued to *show* us more and more that she was not a sick child. One of the things we pride ourselves on over the years is how hard we worked *not* to think of, or treat her, like a sick child. Sure, people stared at the feeding tube wherever we went. But we stopped caring after awhile, and Jaclyn was too young to notice stares from strangers.

Jaclyn's speech wasn't progressing as early as I would have liked. But I accepted that she might be delayed in many developmental areas. Plus, she had that feeding tube down her throat, and while nobody could tell me with certainty whether it might affect her speech, I worried that it had. Just before turning two, she uttered her first word: "Ball." For so long, this child had been taking in her surroundings because she was immobile and could do little else. The beginning of speech came slowly, but once she started talking she never stopped.

Our days were filled with tube feedings and the logistics of eating and reflux. When we weren't engulfed in the whole eating routine, Jaclyn was in speech and physical therapy. I have to admit that, over time, I slacked off when it came to practicing at home what we learned in therapy. Jaclyn wouldn't cooperate with me and allow me to move her body (for physical therapy) or to stimulate her mouth (for speech therapy) as she did for actual therapists. Exercising at home was frustrating. I was also exhausted. So I didn't do much of it. Instead, I did what I knew how to do, and what I could be successful at: I worked to help stimulate her mind.

When we were home, we tackled sedentary projects head-on. I continued reading to her. She would sit on the floor and look through books by herself, often repeating the stories that she had memorized. She was funny to listen to and to watch. We also made crafts, all kinds of crafts. We made bookmarks out of popsicle sticks and decorated them with sequins and glitter. We made pencil holders from empty soup cans and glued dry pasta noodles or wrapping paper all over them. We made these projects for ourselves and enough to give away to relatives too. Jaclyn had her hands in fingerpaint, Play-Doh, and clay more than I care to remember those days. My mom made papier maché for us to play with too. We blew bubbles in the house. It was therapeutic, and it was fun. And we did puzzles. Boy, did we do puzzles.

Jaclyn was a toddler when we started playing computer games. I bought or borrowed library disks for toddlers. We would sit and play games that taught shapes, numbers, letters, and even Spanish. Her attention span was amazing, and she took in information easily. We also started to play board games—*Candyland, Chutes and Ladders, Go Fish, Hi Ho Cherry-O, Concentration,* and *Memory*. Jaclyn learned game rules and new strategies easily. Her love of board games began as a toddler and continued with a vengeance!

Jaclyn loved to make pictures. She put stickers all over paper, and she loved to color. She always used bright colors. The first time I painted her toenails and fingernails with polish made her laugh and laugh. As she got older, it was not unusual for her to request different colors of nail polish for each finger—a rainbow—or to have me paint stripes on her nails. Her personality was bright and colorful too.

Over time, we got more adventurous and left the house more. I started taking her to museums, mostly because we were becoming bored at home. I took her to the zoo and for long walks around the neighborhood. We watched ducks swim in ponds. We went to the library every week—something we never tired of! We took a music class. We went to the park. But being at the playground was not an easy experience, for either Jaclyn or for me. She still couldn't climb easily, and ladders were impossible for her to master. She had barely any strength in her little legs and butt, which made climbing a single ladder step all but impossible. I had to climb with her. I walked the playground planks with her and carried her through the tunnels. We slid down slides with her on my lap. She enjoyed playing in the sandbox. She could sit in a baby swing by herself, and while pushing her back and forth, I taught her the ABCs.

Other mothers at the park could sit and chat. Their children were safe enough to play unassisted. Going to the park for me was truly tiring. I never established the camaraderie that the other moms had developed with each other, and I was jealous. But then again, maybe I shouldn't have wanted that so desperately because often these were the parents whose children could say the rudest things. "What's coming out of her nose?" "Why do you have to carry her up the ladder if she's not a baby?" Or my "favorite" question, "What's **wrong** with her?"

By now I had learned to brush off insensitive comments. I had Jaclyn on a tube-feeding schedule, with therapy interspersed during the week. We were homebodies a lot, but my mom was living with us for weeks at a time in between her trips back to California. Various aunts and cousins came over to visit us regularly too. We filled the time. We played together. We laughed together. We made projects together. We enjoyed each other totally and completely. It was time to gear up for more changes.

Lessons Jaclyn Taught Me.

Find fun, no matter how difficult that might be. It's very easy to get bogged down with the complexities of a medical condition. But Jaclyn was so much more than her heart condition! I learned from this vivacious child that my own exhaustion and stress were not an excuse to deny finding the time and energy to play with her.

It's Time to Start Doing Things Other People Do

In spite of all the craziness of surgeries and illness, we did manage to make great memories those first years. For instance, we traveled with Jaclyn to visit my mom and brother in California. The amount of medical equipment that had to be transported with us was a bit overwhelming, but we did it. Not only did people stare at Jaclyn's feeding tube, but also at the oxygen she needed while in flight. Most people's bodies can compensate for the slight decrease in oxygen that is experienced while in a plane. But because Jaclyn's normal oxygen levels even after surgery were just over 90%, a drop in oxygen brought her to 80%. This could make breathing more difficult and labored so, to fly, Jaclyn required supplemental oxygen.

Logistically, arranging for oxygen on a plane required a round of phone calls. When Jaclyn was older and we had flown more often with her, we became experts in the whole process. Sometimes flight attendants had little or no knowledge of the oxygen system, and therefore we often set the oxygen tank accordingly. Not a problem—we knew what to do.

In order to have oxygen on a plane, an oxygen tank would be stored in the overhead compartment. A tube comes out of the bin and would be taped to the ceiling above Jaclyn's seat. As if the dangling tubing wasn't enough to cause stares, seeing the cannula in Jaclyn's nose often did. Jaclyn took this all in stride.

Another hassle was the medical equipment that we had to bring with us when we flew. None of our equipment could be packed in luggage for fear of damage. Instead, it had to be carried on the plane with us. This required careful packing and extended time in security while personnel checked each piece of equipment. When Jaclyn was little, we had to bring the oximeter, Kangaroo pump, and also her nebulizer, used for breathing treatments when she had respiratory infections. All three pieces of equipment had motors in them, a big red flag to airport security, which further delayed our travels.

While there were difficulties involved in traveling with Jaclyn when she was young, it was worth it because it created memories of a "normal" childhood. Another example of trying to do normal things was when we decided to buy a larger home. We saw a new development being built and jumped at the chance to have a bigger house. We busied ourselves with all the details, but besides it being a hectic time, it was also exciting. During that period, we were able to temporarily "forget" about illness and focus instead on some of the mundane things that other people did, like picking floor trim and deciding where to put windows.

Another issue we had been postponing was potty-training. Jaclyn was ready, but her diuretics made it difficult. However, we pushed forward, and in two days she was out of diapers. She quickly mastered staying dry all night too, but as soon as she awoke in the morning, she needed to race to the bathroom. If there was any delay, she would have accidents, which upset her terribly. She was, after all, trying to be a "big girl." It wasn't her fault that she needed diuretics, so we were constantly on vigil to hear her in order to avoid this problem.

But the biggest issue that Alan and I had put off because of surgeries and hospitalizations had been about when to have another child. It didn't seem like there was a right time, knowing Jaclyn had so many procedures and surgeries coming up. In our one-time ideal world, I had wanted our children to be two years apart. But when Jaclyn was younger and had more closely scheduled surgeries, it didn't seem reasonable to have another baby. Eventually I realized that life with Jaclyn meant we were never done with procedures and surgeries. So we took the plunge and considered having another baby.

Even though Jaclyn's cardiac anomalies were not genetic, a "fluke of nature" as the doctors explained, I had earlier insisted on further testing. Alan, Jaclyn and I had undergone genetic testing when Jaclyn was an infant. The results confirmed there was no genetic basis for Jaclyn's heart's development, so now we forged ahead with plans for another child. I got pregnant right away.

This time I was labeled as a "high risk pregnancy" simply because there was no explanation for Jaclyn's irregular heart development. Being high risk meant many things. For one, it meant that I was poked and prodded a lot. I had an amniocentesis and anxiously awaited the results, which confirmed a healthy pregnancy. The high risk label also translated into appointments with a perinatal cardiologist to look at the development of the baby's heart in utero, and also a perinatologist to check for other birth defects. I was quite relieved when both doctors pointed out the developing pulmonary artery in this baby. All was going well.

At some point during my pregnancy, it was decided that Jaclyn would need her fourth surgery soon, also open-heart. We didn't want to wait until after our second child was born, because he/she wouldn't be allowed to be with us in the PSHU with Jaclyn. And we didn't want to leave a newborn at home with a babysitter while in the hospital with Jaclyn for weeks on end. So we scheduled the surgery for April, 1999, a month before Jaclyn's third birthday. I was due in mid-June. As usual, it was a precarious time for us.

Lessons Jaclyn Taught Me.

Forge ahead with the business of living. It would have been easy to let Jaclyn's heart condition take over our lives. Over the years, we have met families with chronically ill children whose lives often revolved around illness. We realized early on that putting off vacations, moving, having other children, or anything for that matter, was an easy trap to fall into. Certainly there were long stretches of time when we were focused on a surgery or a recovery and nothing else. During those times we operated in "medical mode." But we also learned to make plans and move forward when we were between medical procedures. Plans could always be changed if a medical necessity arose, but our living didn't have to stop.

Gearing Up For Round Four

As the fourth surgery neared, we shifted into "medical mode." This meant putting ourselves into quarantine again, or the closest thing to it, in order to keep Jaclyn healthy. Prior to both the third and fourth surgeries, Jaclyn had to undergo cardiac catheterizations. These procedures were scheduled weeks before each surgery. A catheter would be inserted through an artery into her groin and fished up to her heart. Pictures would be taken and venous pressures would be measured in her heart and lung vessels. Each catheterization necessitated an overnight hospital stay. And each one left a small scar along her bikini line.

Jaclyn was now almost three years old and very bright and curious. She was old enough to understand more about what was to come. We explained to her that after surgery she would wake up with a tube in her mouth and throat and that she wouldn't be able to talk to us. She hated IVs, especially because of the maddening amounts of tape nurses used to secure them. The worst part for Jaclyn was having her arm taped to a board, all the way from her fingers to just above the elbow. This was done so the IV wouldn't loosen or come out when she bent her arm or wrist. Consequently, she couldn't bend her arm for the duration of the stay in the hospital; she found this terribly uncomfortable and annoying.

Keeping Jaclyn and our house germ-free was very difficult and stressful. But we did it. Other than Alan and me, we didn't let anyone in or out of our house (except when Alan absolutely had to go to his office). Upon returning from work, he immediately washed his hands in the bathroom beside the garage. Family members again delivered groceries to our house, and Jaclyn and I simply stayed put. The surgery took place in April, 1999. After three previous surgeries, one might think that we, as parents, would have had a better handle on what to expect. But, once again, I found myself caught off-guard by what Jaclyn looked like after surgery.

Doctors, nurses, and surgeons do a lot to prepare parents for surgery, including explaining potential risks. But the after-surgery facts, like being told that your child will have tubes and wires coming out of virtually every part of her/his tiny body, are often not discussed. There were IVs in both arms and a triple lumen (or central line) in her groin, which was actually three IVs going into three holes in the same area. There was, of course, a ventilator, a chest tube, a catheter, and various additional pumps and syringes of medicine being put into our child. The amount of medical equipment leading to Jaclyn's body right after surgery has always been astounding to me. There was also the large incision, which post-surgery looked oozy, bloody and swollen. The whole thought of a scalpel making that mark upsets me terribly.

We were unprepared for the various marks all over Jaclyn's body after surgery. Some of these marks included irritated skin from various tapes used on her during surgery. I later found out that Jaclyn's eyes were taped shut in the operating room, thus explaining the puffy eyes. She was also covered with miscellaneous bruises from failed IVs or from catheters that were to be put into veins or arteries but, due to scarring from previous surgeries, were no longer usable. The bottom line was that after surgery, Jaclyn, and probably most children who have been through what she had, looked like hell.

When she opened her eyes the first time after surgery, we were beside her, as we had promised to be. She was still on a ventilator, so when she tried to cry no sound came out. She was scared.

These are the things I wish I had been told. Granted, there is much information the surgeon and doctors need to dispense. But sometimes it was the "little" things that put me over the edge, simply because I didn't anticipate them.

This fourth surgery proved to be the most difficult recovery for Jaclyn. Her body took on fluids again, she required blood transfusions, she spiked fevers, and she constantly fought the ventilator. We tried to explain to our child to stop thrashing around in her bed and to stop trying to cry/scream/talk so it would not hurt so much. But she was only three! She didn't understand. At that point, we didn't either. While her lungs recovered, she had to stay on that ventilator. Those days were heart-wrenching to bear.

Finally, after several days, Jaclyn was removed from the ventilator—a cause for celebration. But upon its removal, she wouldn't even look at us. She was angry, and we felt terrible. Despite our attempts to soothe her, stroke her, sing to her, or read to her, she ignored us. Instead, she lay in her ICU bed looking at anything other than our faces. It tore us apart to imagine how much she must have hated us then.

Day after day my husband, mother, aunt, in-laws and I had sat at Jaclyn's bedside, reading to her, watching movies with her, listening to music with her, and talking to her. Finally Jaclyn came around to her old self and would once again look at us. Her voice was high-pitched and raspy from being on the ventilator for close to a week. The days and nights were terribly long. An ICU crib is raised with rails on the sides. Regular chairs aren't high enough to allow a parent to reach in to touch their child, so we sat on stools. But because I was now eight months pregnant, sitting for hours would strain my back, forcing me to take brief walks to stretch. I was terribly uncomfortable but had no choice.

After a few days, Jaclyn was encouraged to try to eat. She was still NG-tube fed. However, a miracle was about to happen. While we prided ourselves on not leaving Jaclyn alone in PSHU, there were moments when we had done just that. For instance, during nurses' shift change, all parents were ordered off the unit. Jaclyn seemed to handle this better than Alan and I did.

However, one time a nurse cajoled us to go and eat while Jaclyn was asleep. We had regularly left Jaclyn with my mom or in-laws while we grabbed some food or showered at the Guest House. But sometime during the third week post-surgery, we felt it would be okay to leave Jaclyn alone for the first time, in the care of her nurse. She was, after all, sleeping. What could happen?

When we returned, Jaclyn was sitting up in bed. Not terribly unusual. However, her nurse, Deborah, was spoon-feeding her baby food. We walked into the room and were simply flabbergasted. Jaclyn had not eaten food before by mouth. She was three years old. She then proceeded to ask for a drink. Deborah held a regular cup for her, and to our amazement, Jaclyn drank it. Again, she had never had a drink by mouth before. She had been tube-fed all this time. We couldn't believe what we were seeing, yet it was true—our daughter had finally mastered eating and drinking.

There was only one problem—Jaclyn was on fluid restrictions, so she could not eat or drink at her leisure. We could only give her drips of apple juice or grape juice. We wanted to let her drink a gallon, just so she would realize how good it was and to remember how to do it! We could only give her tiny rations of the foods which were considered liquids and therefore restricted. This was pure torture for us. Here was our child, eating and drinking for the first time, and we couldn't let her have what she wanted, when she wanted it. We will never forget Deborah, not only for her attempts to feed Jaclyn, but also for her persistence in making it happen. To have it be a surprise for us was truly a gift!

Suddenly, I had a mission. I bought one jar of every kind of baby food I could find at the Kmart down the street from the hospital. I wanted Jaclyn to experience tastes. She had gone without taste for such a long time that I was thrilled to offer her a selection. But no matter what we tried, she seemed to prefer the same few fruity baby foods—applesauce, peaches, pears, plums, and Blueberry Buckle.

I have fond memories of Blueberry Buckle. It's a Gerber Stage Three baby food that is rather thick and purple, and it turned out to be Jaclyn's favorite. By the end of our hospital stay, everybody on the unit knew that Jaclyn had reached a major milestone—eating—and everybody knew that she preferred Blueberry Buckle to everything else.

To help pass the long three-week period we were spending in ICU, my mom and I embarked on a project. How do you thank the many nurses and doctors who have cared for your child? It's almost impossible to extend appreciation. So we began to hand-paint picture frames for each nurse who had cared for Jaclyn. We took turns playing with Jaclyn and coming out to the family waiting room to paint. My husband, as well as other families sharing that space, thought we were insane. On the waiting room floor, we spread out our frames, sand paper, brushes, and paints. We painted throughout the days and nights, making these thank you gifts to distribute upon discharge. Each was colorful, whimsical and unique. And Jaclyn designated which frame went to which nurse and doctor.

Nearing the end of our hospital stay, I was eight months pregnant. Each set-back Jaclyn would experience would bring countless nurses to my side, with fears that I would go into premature labor. I endured blood pressure checks throughout Jaclyn's stay. I was fine and would be ecstatic when Jaclyn was discharged, days shy of her third birthday.

This fourth surgery kept Jaclyn in the hospital for 24 days. And her recovery was still not over. We were told she would probably not need another surgery until she was around ages six to eight, depending on growth spurts. Three to five years away from the hospital sounded like heaven!

"Normalcy" Sets in Yet Again

We were in the middle of Jaclyn's recovery, I was about to have our second child, and we were also building a house—all at the same time. We received an offer on our old house the day Jaclyn came off the ventilator. Alan worked out the details of the sale from a phone in the hospital hallway.

Once we came home from the hospital, I channeled my nervous energy into planning a birthday party for Jaclyn. Looking back now it was ridiculous to undertake a large birthday celebration at that time with all the craziness in our lives. But I was determined that Jaclyn have the party she so deserved.

Post-surgery, Jaclyn once again needed to be carried up and down the steps. Her breastbone needed four more weeks to fully heal. Her heart also needed to recover. She came home from the hospital on large dosages of multiple medications; the focus of her recovery included weaning her off of these. Moreover, she was weak and unable to climb stairs in our house. Her legs had atrophied. She couldn't even climb into her own bed. It was frustrating to realize how much ground we had lost with her physical therapy. She had lost weight too, which was a huge concern because of how difficult it was for her to consume enough calories in the first place. We were carrying and lifting her a lot. And I was very pregnant, which made it all the more difficult.

Additionally, she was covered with miscellaneous bruises, including dark rings under her eyes. This time there were other effects from surgery, too. Her voice was still high pitched and squeaky from the many days on the ventilator. She sounded like someone who had inhaled helium and then attempted to speak. I was worried this would be her permanent voice because we were told that she could have strained her vocal cords while thrashing about on a ventilator for so many days. I was mortified at the prospect of this. It took eight long months for her voice to return to its normal pitch.

However, it was important for us to keep moving forward. Jaclyn's third birthday party went off without a hitch. Both of our extended families came. But looking back at pictures from the party one can see that Jaclyn really looked like she had been through the ringer!

When Jaclyn returned part-time to the home daycare after this surgery, she was taking a few spoonfuls of baby food. It took a long time to feed her, but at least we felt we were finally moving in the right direction. She was still getting the majority of her nutrition from the feeding tube during the day and at night.

As Jaclyn increased her caloric intake by mouth, Alan and I were encouraged to stop tube feedings. The plan was to see if she would get hungry enough to eat more. This child had never experienced hunger; she had always been fed on a strict schedule. We had tried this numerous times before, with no success. Jaclyn just refused to eat and therefore received no calories. We were encouraged to see how long she would hold out; the longest Alan and I could let her go without eating was two days. She was taking in very few calories by mouth and still wasn't learning to satiate the hunger feeling by eating more.

On the morning of New Year's Eve, Jaclyn accidentally pulled out her feeding tube. We decided that the beginning of a new year was as good a time as any to stop the tube feedings permanently. We bit the bullet. The first few days didn't go well but despite feeling rotten for denying her calories, we pushed it farther. Miraculously, a few days later Jaclyn started consuming more. She wasn't eating nearly as many calories as she was supposed to, but after 2 ½ years of relying on an NG-tube, we were finally done. We had overcome a major obstacle, and there was no going back.

Meanwhile, I had returned to work after having taken off for

Jaclyn's surgery and recovery. I decided to work only two days a week instead of three. My colleagues were very accommodating, but the stress I felt was internal. I didn't feel that I was contributing to my job as much as I wanted to; yet I was constrained by life events. When Jaclyn was sick, Alan and I would take turns staying home with her. However he often traveled for work, and inevitably Jaclyn would be sick when he was out of town or on a day when he had important clients to meet in town. It got to the point where I was embarrassed to tell my colleagues I had to stay home again. While nobody questioned it, I felt guilty.

Furthermore, I was about to have my second baby, so my accommodating workplace would have to bear with me through that too. The difficult part for me was that a colleague was pregnant at the same time I was. She had her baby and was right back to work. I had already taken time off for Jaclyn's surgery, so I felt I didn't dare bring up the notion of time off again following my second child's birth. Seeing how exhausted I was, my supervisor decided that I needed more time to recuperate; he told me to return when I was ready. There would be no pressure from work. The pressure I felt was originating from within.

I wanted to "have it all." It felt great to be at work, to feel useful and good at what I was doing. I loved embarking on new research projects and writing papers. The excitement of having one of my articles accepted for publication in a scholarly journal was a high for me. But I simply wasn't giving it my all—because I couldn't. I was determined, however, to keep it up because I felt I deserved the chance to work and have a family too. Others did it. Other people who had more children than I had were able to do it. Why couldn't I? It just wasn't fair.

In June of 1999, our son Ryan was born. When Jaclyn came to the hospital to meet her baby brother, I had tears in my eyes as she held him on her lap. This child had just undergone major open-heart surgery and was clearly not back to herself in strength or endurance. Yet the pictures we have of Jaclyn smiling and holding her baby brother for the first time are pure treasures! She had been through the mill, but we had somehow survived…again!

With a new baby at home, there was little pressure to go out. Jaclyn, Ryan and I took full advantage of being homebodies. It was a time for Jaclyn to continue healing and also a time to catch up on our rest. Summertime was relaxing and re-energizing. We had certainly been through enough in the past few months, and yet the big moving day into our newly built house was looming. In August, we moved into our new house. It was a fresh start and an exciting time.

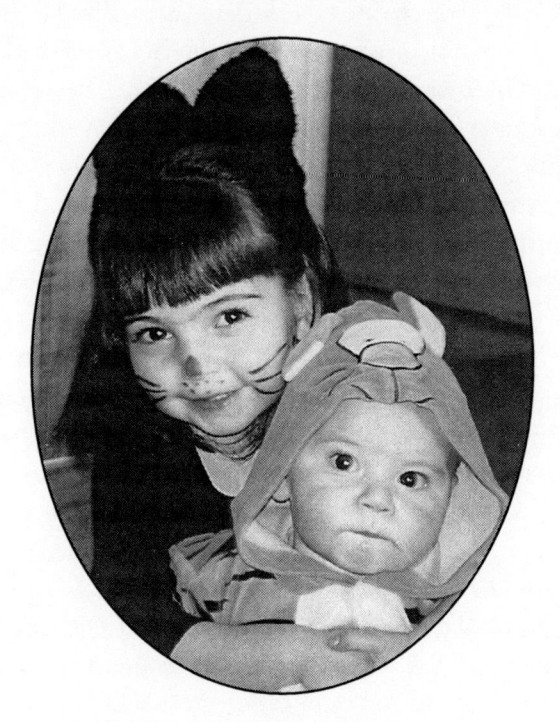

Halloween with Ryan, October, 1999.

    Patterns established early for Jaclyn continued. She was beginning a new adventure at this time: pre-school. The idea of pre-school terrified me, but Jaclyn was almost four years old and it was time. I worried about germs, about her being knocked over, about her becoming tired, and about how others would treat her. There were still many physical feats that she was not capable of, and I was concerned that she would be teased. She had very little arm strength which meant she couldn't open a glue stick, she couldn't push down on a soap dispenser, she couldn't snap her own pants, she couldn't tear off paper towels from a roll, and she had difficulty turning door knobs to open them.

    When Jaclyn entered pre-school, her teachers were concerned

about her frailty, but Jaclyn showed them she had a strong desire to try to keep up with her peers and possessed an air of confidence about her. The teachers were wonderfully patient, and my fears about other kids' comments were, thankfully, unrealistic.

Between the ages of three and four, Jaclyn blossomed in many ways. Her speech and vocabulary sky-rocketed. Her memory was amazing—she remembered the tiniest details. I think that being immobile as an infant made her more observant of the world around her.

She began to hold a pencil and crayons correctly. She colored, but that became boring, for her and for me. So I bought maze books, dot-to-dot books, and workbooks. She had difficulty getting her pencil to maneuver through mazes, but she could clearly grasp the concept of what she was supposed to do. Though not always neat, she was awfully good at all these activities. She seemed to crave learning, and I was more than happy to oblige her! She learned numbers and easily picked up basic addition too. She was not a physical child and often stayed away from rough kinds of play. But she soaked up workbooks and learning. She could write her name early, and she soon began to spell words too. She liked to make my grocery lists for me, and it was always fun to read her inventive spelling.

Even bath time was a time for learning. Although she had all kinds of bath toys, the ones she preferred most were letters of the alphabet that stuck to the tub wall. This is how she started to learn her sounds, and she wanted to practice every night. She was truly taking in anything I offered her, and she couldn't seem to get enough. It was very exciting. Her mind was so sharp. This was why I worried about risks to her brain from surgeries, and it is why I prayed for "no disabling disabilities."

At some point I realized that the physical conquests would either come someday for Jaclyn or perhaps they wouldn't, but the cognitive component needed to be constantly stimulated too. Maybe I shouldn't have been so focused on it, but as long as she was still getting physical therapy, and by age four also occupational therapy, the learning component was the area into which I channeled a greater portion of my time and energy.

From the time Jaclyn was born, we used to visit my grandmother, Nanny. She was home-bound and always loved the

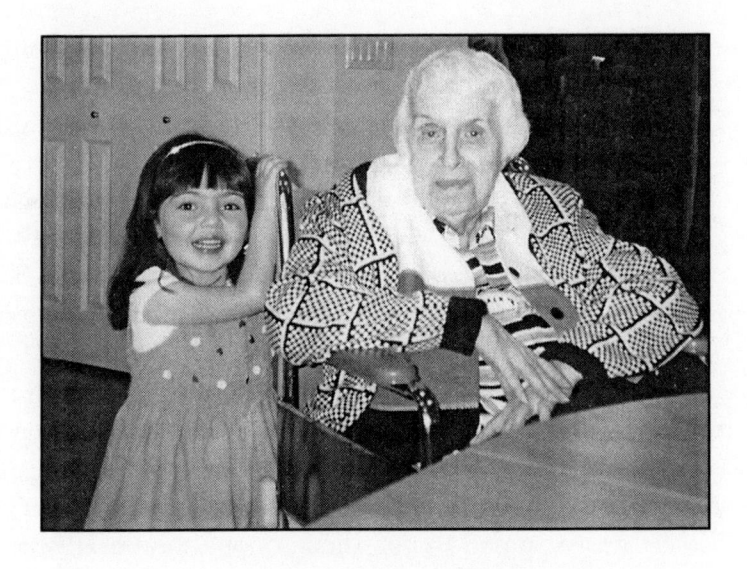

Jaclyn with Nanny (great grandmother).

company. Nanny was an avid reader and card-player. She had a wooden lap board that lay across her armchair so she could pay bills, write letters, read, and do word search puzzles. By the time Jaclyn was three or four, she would stand beside Nanny's chair to play cards. *Old Maid* turned into *Go Fish*, which years later became *Gin Rummy*, *Blackjack* and *Canasta*. Jaclyn loved this attention and fun. As she got older, Jaclyn liked buying new word search puzzle books for her great-grandmother. When Nanny died years later, in 2003, Jaclyn kept Nanny's lap board and her two favorite decks of cards. The lapboard still sits beside Jaclyn's bed as she often used it at night to do her own word search puzzles before going to sleep.

Lessons Jaclyn Taught Me.

Illness can be compartmentalized. Surely there are times when illness can be all-consuming. But other times, chronic illness deserves little attention in one's day-to-day life. Find a way to do "normal" things in spite of illness. Jaclyn wouldn't have it any other way.

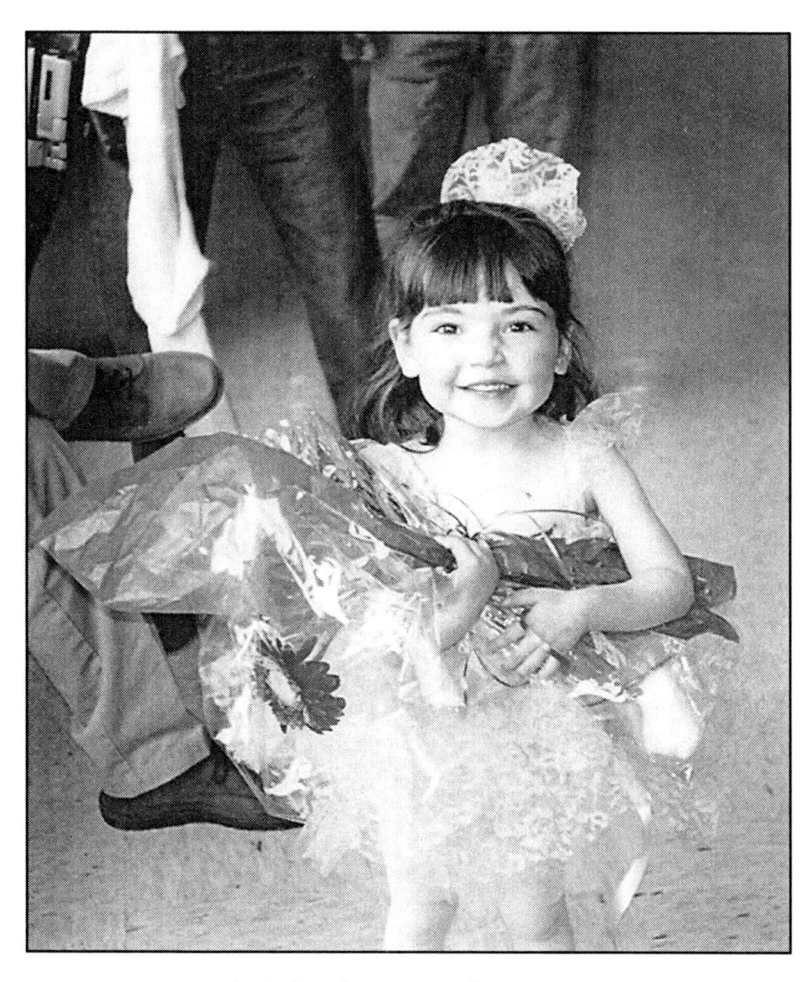

Jaclyn's first dance recital, May, 2000.

The Second Child Feels Like a First

With Ryan's birth came a whole new set of emotions. I was excited and overjoyed; he was adorable, sweet, easy, and fun. However, at times I couldn't help looking at him and seeing all the things Jaclyn and I had missed.

When Ryan was born, my mom sold her house in California and moved back to Chicago—about seven miles from our house. She missed her grandchildren and once again became a tremendous help to me.

From the time Ryan started to hold his head up, general developmental milestones took on added importance. We hadn't had many of the expected milestones with Jaclyn, so this was new to us. I used to spend hours watching Ryan roll, reach, rock, crawl, move, eat, pull himself up, stand, and climb. Basic movement was so easy for him. Nothing was a struggle. He moved with grace, in ways that Jaclyn never could. For instance, he could lean over to pick up something that had fallen. By itself this was not very exciting. In contrast, when Jaclyn dropped something, or an item was out of her grasp, she sat patiently waiting for someone to retrieve it. She was not physically able to move from her spot to get it, and simply didn't try. Ryan, on the other hand, let nothing stand in his way; he had a full range of motion and motivation, which kept him moving constantly.

When Jaclyn was a baby, I used to lay her on blankets on my bathroom floor with an activity center above her while I took morning showers. Once she could sit up, I'd prop her around pillows, but she'd inevitably fall over and not be able to get back to a sitting position. Because her first two surgeries cut through muscles under her arms, she wasn't able to roll to one side, bear weight on her arms, or use her stomach and arm muscles to push herself to a sitting position. Instead she stayed lying down. If she fell onto pillows while I was in the shower, I would jump out to sit her up again. After a while, I realized I could safely prop her in the middle of my king-size bed, surrounded by pillows, with the television on, while I took my quick shower. Other mothers gasped at the notion that I left an infant alone on a bed while out of the room. But I was sure that she could not, in any possible way, fall off that bed. If she were to fall over from sitting, she'd simply be stuck on the pillows around her. She couldn't roll off the bed. She couldn't crawl off the bed. She couldn't move. I could take a quick shower without worry.

With Ryan, on the other hand, barricades of any kind were never enough. He got into everything—all the time. I was as unprepared regarding his sense of movement as a first time parent might have been.

For me, Ryan provided constant entertainment but at the same time, a sense of longing. I would look at him, laugh at him, play with him, chase him, love him, and realize all that Jaclyn had missed. I also saw that at age three and then four, she still didn't move with ease. Her struggles were more pronounced at these ages, simply because I now had a means of comparison.

Six weeks after Ryan was born, I returned to my part-time work. Ryan and Jaclyn went to the home daycare on my work days, and Jaclyn attended pre-school two days a week. We were on a different schedule. This "normalcy" felt good.

My Needs Become Secondary

While all moms probably experience losing a sense of themselves to a child to some extent, it was especially hard for me to focus on my own needs when Jaclyn required so much. For many years, I simply thought of my needs as unimportant.

Even when Jaclyn was eating on her own and tube-feeding was over, I still had a rigorous schedule to follow with her. For instance, her medications had to be timed just right for many reasons. Some medications had to be taken apart from others because, together, they could cause a severe drop in her blood pressure. However, they both had to be given in the morning before school. So it was imperative for me to be sure she got the first medication on time, so the second one would not be delayed, making her late for school. Also, some of her medications were given multiple times during the day. One was given three times per day; therefore, each dose needed to be about eight hours apart. For a child, it is almost impossible to separate medications appropriately without waking her during the night to do it.

Jaclyn was on six medications a day for about five years. The schedule looked like this: At 7:00 am, I syringed a diuretic, Lasix, into her mouth while she was asleep. By the time she was awake, the diuretic would be working, and she would race to the bathroom. Around 7:45 am (or whenever she would wake up), she would receive a bronchial inhaler. Between 8:00 am and 8:30 am, she received two liquid medications with breakfast—Captopril for her heart pressures and Spironolactone, another diuretic. Then she would go to school. After school Jaclyn would have her second dose of Spironolactone and the second of three doses of Captopril. These would be given with a snack because they required food. Before dinner she would have her second dose of Lasix and a dose of Tracleer, a medication for pulmonary arterial hypertension. Between 6:30 and 7:00 pm, she would get Digoxin, a heart medication. When she would brush her teeth for bed, she would have her inhaler again. Finally, before he went to bed, Alan would give Jaclyn's third dose of Captopril. It had to be given approximately eight hours after the late afternoon dose. He was able to syringe this liquid into Jaclyn's mouth while she was sleeping because she learned how to swallow without being awakened.

If we were not going to be home during the day or evening, we had to bring medicines with us. Some of Jaclyn's medications were light-sensitive, meaning they could not be exposed to light or they would be ineffective. This required us to either take the whole bottle with us or to take the proper amount in a capped syringe that was tightly wrapped in a paper towel and sealed with a rubber band. Other medications required refrigeration so we packed them in an insulated bag with an ice pack. Over time, we easily adapted to Jaclyn's medication schedule. I knew what time it was at any given moment of any day, in order to know what she needed and if I needed to pack it with us. After awhile, her medication schedule was just something I handled without thinking about it; I did it because I had to.

Another example of how my needs felt unimportant had to do with little things I simply didn't address for myself. For instance, the woman who cuts my hair used to tease me about how long I could wait between cuts. When Jaclyn was little, I would sometimes go for days without wearing makeup and hardly ever wore jewelry. These were simple things. They didn't require much time on my part, but when your child has so many needs, each day tends to be focused on him/her.

When she was still an infant, I would get up in the morning and immediately be on alert for Jaclyn to awaken. Having been fed all night via Kangaroo pump, she would have a full stomach. And crying out for attention often was accompanied by reflux vomiting. Sometimes her NG-tube would come out and would lie across her tongue, causing her to gag and choke. I couldn't possibly be in the shower or be drying my hair during these times because then I wouldn't hear her. So it was just easier for me to wake up in the morning, take record-breaking speed showers, and throw on some clothes (minus much attention to hair, makeup or jewelry).

After Jaclyn was born, I lost my pregnancy weight rather quickly. I lost additional weight too, to the point that my pre-pregnancy clothes were too big. My mother used to offer to stay with Jaclyn so I could do errands, such as shop for myself, but I didn't have the energy or the desire. It just didn't seem important.

I recall how judgmental I was of people who spent time pampering themselves. Time away from their children. Time doing things solely for themselves.

I also felt envious of friends and family members who traveled for work and pleasure. I knew they worked hard, but leaving their children home for long periods with babysitters, even grandparents, made me extremely jealous. I think I was longing for the professional life I had given up, but also the couple relationship that we were not able to have because of her needs. Before Jaclyn was born, Alan and I had gone out most weekends. But with Jaclyn's medical needs, a regular babysitter was out of the question. My mom was almost our exclusive babysitter when Jaclyn was an infant and toddler. When she was in town, she stayed with Jaclyn so Alan and I could go on "dates" together. As Jaclyn got older, my in-laws and aunt and uncle also took care of Jaclyn, but no one except my mom could re-insert the feeding tube if it came out.

By the time Ryan was a toddler, things had settled down a bit with Jaclyn's needs. She was healed, eating on her own, and the "repair" of her heart had been completed with four surgeries. Ryan was content to play by himself for hours! With Jaclyn in pre-school two mornings a week and Ryan entertaining himself with books, blocks, or any toy with wheels, I found some free time during the day for myself. I started calling friends from college and graduate school, friends who were also home with their kids. I called for no other reason than to chat. I had not done this for years. I began hand-painting frames to sell. I started reading again, something I had always loved but didn't have time to do. Even being at work part-time and travelling once a year to professional conferences were indulgences for me.

As Jaclyn and Ryan got older, I became better about tending

to my own needs. I can more easily tell my kids that I need quiet time—to read or talk on the phone without feeling guilty. I've come a long way, mostly because Jaclyn's needs eased over time. But the patterns set when she was younger, that many parents who deal with chronic illness get stuck in, definitely took a while to break.

When one feels one's needs are secondary, it is not easy to realize that at some point life *will* get better or easier. "Someday" is an indefinite time and can make one feel trapped. Countless people assured me that things *would* get better, but I didn't see a light at the end of the tunnel. I didn't know when Jaclyn would need me less, but eventually she did. Through a combination of her health improving, and my persistence in making my own needs important again, it did happen. Life got easier.

Lessons Jaclyn Taught Me.

Trust your feelings regarding your child's care. Until Jaclyn was about three years old, leaving her with anyone other than Alan or my mother was uncomfortable for me. My needs *were* in fact secondary to hers. I didn't resent Jaclyn or the situation; it was just simply the way it was. And no matter what anyone told me, I wouldn't waver from this viewpoint.

When Jaclyn's health improved, I did begin making time for myself. She taught me to trust my intuition and not care what others told me was the "right" thing to do. There was no right or wrong way to live, nor was there a script to follow regarding how to care for her. My perspective about what was important—my child—was more important than tending to my own needs.

School Begins

Jaclyn was totally ready to be a kindergartner. The public school is across the field that is in my backyard. I can see the school clearly from my patio doors. Fortunately our school is the smallest one in the district; there are only two classes per grade, and each class has no more than about twenty-three students. Almost every family knows every other family, at least on some level.

Jaclyn couldn't wait to go to school each day. I'd open her blinds in the morning and say, "Good morning, Sunshine. Time to get up and ready for school." She got up easily and dressed herself in the clothes she had carefully chosen the night before. The majority of her clothes were multi-colored or bright, rainbow colors, just the way she liked them. She loved colorful barrettes and ponytail holders too. Jaclyn bounded down to the kitchen for breakfast, anxious and excited for kindergarten every day (and subsequent school years too).

School meant new things to us. Jaclyn now had a chance to be a regular kid. I was adamant about her not being treated as "sick." I met the kindergarten teacher the first week to update her about Jaclyn's needs. I explained that if Jaclyn needed to use the restroom, she really needed to be excused from class right away. Diuretics can wreak havoc on school schedules. I also informed the teacher that Jaclyn would require help opening snacks and juice boxes and lifting her chair on and off the desk at the beginning and end of the school day. No problem.

Kindergarten was a place for Jaclyn to excel. And she did. She was reading early in the school year, she was writing beautifully, and she could spell well from an early age. She also loved math and solved problems in her head. She couldn't wait to do her homework. I used to laugh when she would come home from school and say, "Mom, can I do my homework now?" She couldn't get enough of school and learning, so I continued to supplement her with workbooks and enrolled her in a Spanish class.

It was during kindergarten that we began to use games to challenge Jaclyn even more. We started to play *Monopoly Junior* and she learned how to calculate change. When we played *Yahtzee Junior* she practiced addition. *Boggle Junior* helped her sound out words and spell. With *Scrabble Junior* she mastered letter and word patterns. She could look at a word and tell us how she could make a new word by replacing one particular letter. *Clue Junior* and *Battleship* were other favorite games that taught her how to strategize and solve puzzles.

Because she was in a public school, various therapies that were deemed "educationally relevant" were provided for Jaclyn, free of charge. She qualified for both physical therapy (PT) and occupational therapy (OT). The school also supplied an adaptive physical education (PE) teacher to accompany and assist Jaclyn in gym class.

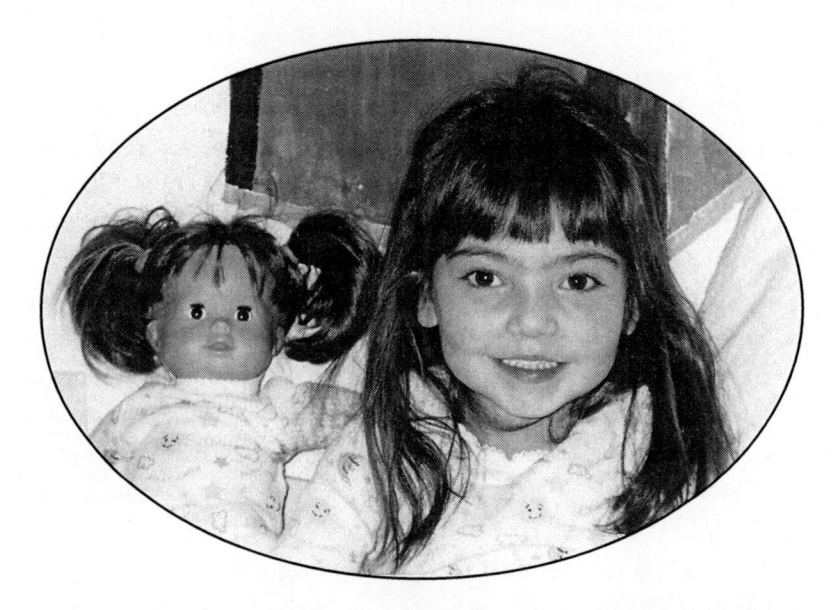

Jaclyn and her doll, Alex, in matching pajamas, March, 2001.

In kindergarten, I met all the therapists. I was told that Jaclyn would receive two twenty-minute periods of PT each week, and one session of OT. PT aimed to increase her general strength and endurance, while OT targeted fine motor skills. In addition to being weak and lacking strength, Jaclyn had difficulty opening bottles, turning doorknobs, unlatching seatbelts, and snapping snaps. The tips of her fingers were somewhat bluish in color, from poor circulation to her extremities, which we assumed contributed to her difficulties.

I was initially told that PT and OT would take place during the school day. But kindergarten was less than three hours, and I didn't want Jaclyn pulled out of class. While I was assured that other children were pulled out for various reasons, I insisted that therapy not interfere with class time. I became Jaclyn's advocate early on—a position I did not waiver from as she got older.

Jaclyn saw the physical therapist one day a week after school. Her second session each week was during recess, which was a very trying period of the day for her anyway. Jaclyn couldn't do some of the things other kids did on the playground, and she was fearful of being knocked over by more active children. Therapy during recess one day each week was a good compromise.

Sometime during the school year, the physical therapist's schedule changed, and she could no longer meet during recess. Instead, she arranged to pull Jaclyn from class without my knowledge. Unfortunately, Jaclyn was missing the time each week that the "gifted teacher" came in to challenge the class with more difficult math problems. Half the school year passed before I had even heard of this gifted teacher's visits and her worksheets. I only found out by chance, when another mom asked me what I thought of the challenging math. I didn't know what she was talking about. I was livid when I found out that Jaclyn had been missing this, as the worksheets were just the kind of added math stimulation Jaclyn craved! I went to school and made sure PT didn't interfere with class time again. Once more I had to use my voice on my child's behalf. As a parent of a chronically ill child, I had a lot on my plate at any given time. Being "on guard" for Jaclyn in this capacity was just one more exhausting and frustrating ordeal that was part of my life.

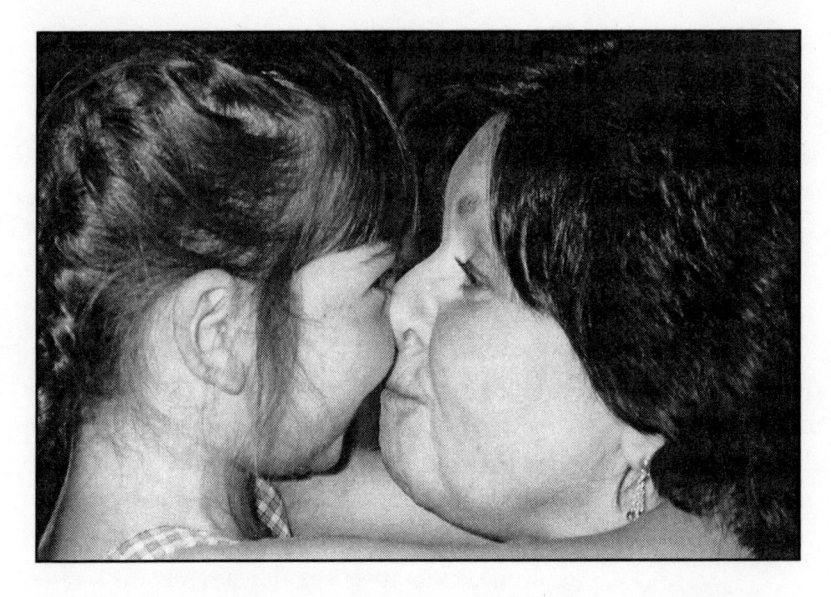

Jaclyn and Mema 'giving Eskimo kisses,' Summer, 2001.

Kindergarten was an experience in which Jaclyn blossomed. She loved school. She made friends easily and invited boys and girls to our house often. When asked what she liked the most about school, Jaclyn always answered "math." When asked, "what do you like the least?" she replied, "recess."

Lessons Jaclyn Taught Me.

Figure out what your child needs and do whatever you must to make that happen. I knew from Jaclyn's love of learning that she needed academic challenges. We used games at home to supplement her craving for new learning. We got ahead in academics and also had fun. One of the smartest decisions I made was insisting that Jaclyn not be pulled from kindergarten to attend physical or occupational therapies. This meant that Jaclyn would not miss precious classroom instruction, thereby being labeled (by herself and by others) as "sick." I believe this contributed immensely to her strong sense of self-esteem.

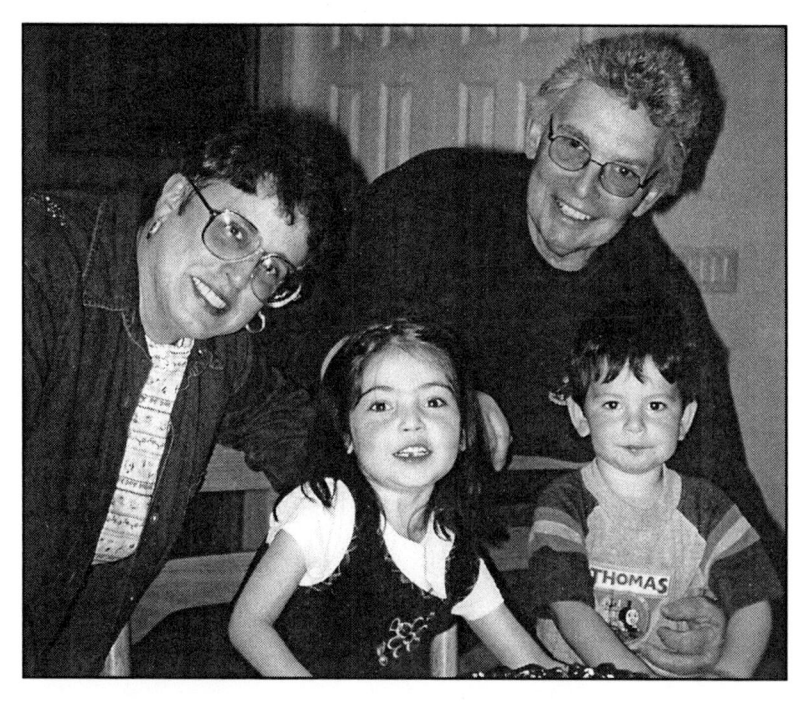

Grandma Bobbi and Grandpa Bob with Jaclyn and Ryan.

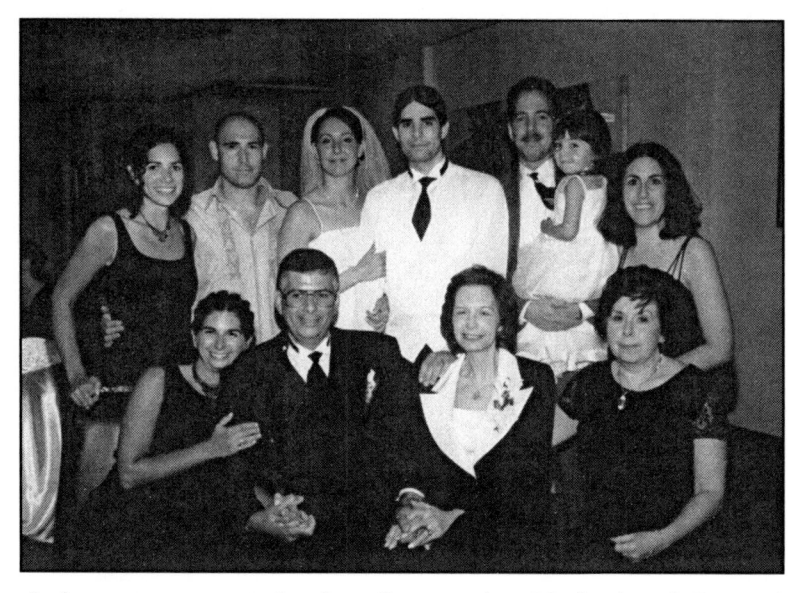

Jaclyn was very excited to be a flower girl in Michael and Corinne's wedding, June, 2001. (Front row: Cousin Jennifer, Uncle Alex, Auntie Karen, Mema. Back row: Cousin Traci, Uncle Danny, Cousin Corinne, Cousin Michael, Daddy, Jaclyn, Me.)

An Extra Bonus Surgery

One month before kindergarten ended and just before Jaclyn turned six years old, she started to complain of stomach aches. They occurred primarily at night, and at first we brushed them off as attempts to postpone bedtime. Jaclyn was a night owl! But after a few days we began to get concerned. The pain was not affecting her eating or her activity level, but as soon as she would lie down in her bed, she would tell us her tummy hurt.

The pediatrician found nothing wrong, but suggested that we adapt Jaclyn's diet. By now Jaclyn's eating had improved to the point that she ate regular food—very small quantities and minimal variety, but better than the earlier days. She was short and thin, but she was eating. The doctor suggested eliminating dairy from her diet, in case she had developed an intolerance to lactose. This was almost impossible for us, since the majority of Jaclyn's calories came from dairy foods—whole milk in large quantities, cheese, yogurt, ice cream, pudding, and butter. Her food repertoire was very slim, so eliminating these foods even for a few days was very difficult. But we tried. Dairy did not seem to be the culprit.

Phone calls to the cardiologist brought no new answers either. We knew that Jaclyn retained fluids, and that her liver often pushed on her stomach. However, that should not have caused the pain she was experiencing to the degree she was feeling it. Every night she was crying that her stomach hurt. After about a week, I took her to see the cardiologist, just to be sure there was nothing anyone was missing. No explanations.

The next visit was to the pediatrician again. After finding nothing medically to explain the pain, the doctor asked us to consider whether this was a ploy for attention, especially since it was confined to bedtime. Alan and I briefly toyed with the idea that psychologically Jaclyn might be trying to control us with talk of pain. However, we did not think this possibility was real because her pain seemed genuine.

More days passed. We spent the nights soothing Jaclyn to sleep, as the pain was still only occurring when she was in bed. Another appointment was made with the pediatrician, mostly because we didn't know what else to do. The doctor told us the only unexamined explanation was the gall bladder. It sounded preposterous that Jaclyn could have gall bladder problems, especially because the pediatrician explained that pain from gall stones could be excruciating. Jaclyn was not in agony, or at least we didn't think so. She was just telling us her tummy hurt.

The pediatrician sent us to the hospital for tests. Sure enough, I got a phone call a few hours later telling me that Jaclyn had calcified gall stones and that her gall bladder needed to be removed. I couldn't believe it. Apparently, it is not uncommon for people to develop calcified stones after they have been on heart/lung machines. Jaclyn had been on a heart/lung machine for each open-heart surgery. There is also a known link between gall stones and being on large amounts of diuretics for extended periods of time, but it is uncommon for these occurrences in a child.

Friends I know who had previously had gall bladder problems described the pain as being almost unbearable. Jaclyn had been living with this for well over a week. We were considering the possibility that it was a psychological ploy for attention, when she was really in intense pain. That was a wake-up call to us that this child's tolerance for pain was indeed very high. Never again did we discount her words.

We were sent to a gastric surgeon who would perform the surgery. It was suggested that we go to a closer, pediatric hospital, rather than the hospital we always used for cardiac care. I was uncomfortable being at another hospital "just in case" a cardiac complication arose. Jaclyn's gall bladder surgery could not be done laproscopically because her liver was too large. So she had another incision an inch from her belly button and about four inches long, horizontally, across her stomach.

It was May, 2002, and Jaclyn was about to turn six years old. She missed the dance recital she had worked five months to prepare for. Instead, we pretended that her rehearsal was the actual recital. She wore her costume, and we took pictures. She was the only child in costume, and the audience consisted only of Alan and I, but we cheered as if she had been on the stage in front of a large audience. We bought her flowers too.

We had planned her birthday parties—one for her friends at a bowling alley and another at home for family. The family party was rescheduled. We gave Jaclyn the choice of postponing her bowling party or having it even while in pain. She wanted the party, so we forged ahead with it on Sunday as planned. Jaclyn turned six on a Monday, and her gall bladder was removed Tuesday. She also missed the "end of kindergarten" party, which really upset her.

Lessons Jaclyn Taught Me.
Listen! Jaclyn didn't complain…not ever. So when she told us her tummy hurt, we believed her. If we had taken advice suggesting she was asserting some control with talk of pain, we wouldn't have been persistent about further testing. Jaclyn taught me not to doubt her or my own feelings. I knew my child, and I believe other parents know their child's tendencies best too, if they only listen.

Another Lesson Jaclyn Taught Me.
Even discomfort doesn't have to completely stop a child from being a child. Jaclyn begged us to let her attend that dance recital rehearsal, since she knew she'd miss the actual recital. We're so glad we complied because the experience and the pictures we have of that day are great memories for her. Better to remember dancing a little, rather than remembering not dancing at all. The same reasoning applied to her bowling birthday party. Jaclyn insisted she wanted the party, and with the doctor's approval, she bowled with her friends and had a birthday celebration. Obviously, we would have skipped the rehearsal and cancelled the party if Jaclyn couldn't participate or if the doctor recommended it. However, as long as we were within the limits of medical approval, we felt that Jaclyn deserved to have childhood memories.

To Have or Not To Have a Third Child

From the time Ryan was a toddler, I considered whether or not I wanted to have a third child. Jaclyn had been away from hospitals and surgeries for years, and she was doing well. Ryan rolled over when he was supposed to, he crawled, he stood, he reached, he ate, and he got into trouble simply because he was mobile. Moreover, he made us laugh and brought us intense joy. Many of the milestones never came easily to Jaclyn, and some never occurred for her at all. So I thought that having a third child would give me another chance to experience those milestones.

My husband, on the other hand, was not having similar thoughts. In his mind, we had one boy and one girl, and he thought that was enough. He was worried about Jaclyn's lifelong surgeries and how hard that would be on Ryan, yet alone another child. But I couldn't shake the feeling that I needed to go through the whole baby thing one more time. It took a lot of arm-twisting, but I talked my husband into having a third child. We got pregnant when Jaclyn was five, and Ryan was two.

During this pregnancy, I decided to leave my part-time position at the Rush Alzheimer's Disease Center. I felt that three children would keep me busy enough, and with continued care in the future for Jaclyn, it made sense for me to stay at home. I was back to being a full-time mom, and other than a semester of part-time teaching at the University of Chicago years later, I haven't looked back.

Jaclyn really wanted a sister, and Ryan was too young to understand or verbalize his thoughts on the matter. Again I was listed as a high-risk pregnancy and underwent an amniocentesis and prenatal cardiology check-ups. All was fine, and Joshua was born in June, 2002. Jaclyn didn't get the sister, but she didn't seem to care. She was the oldest—a role she loved—and she was very happy.

As soon as Joshua was born, I knew that a boy was the best thing in the world that could have happened to Ryan. Both Jaclyn and Ryan were enamored with Joshua from Day One. Jaclyn immediately began acting like a Big Sister, helping with the new baby whenever

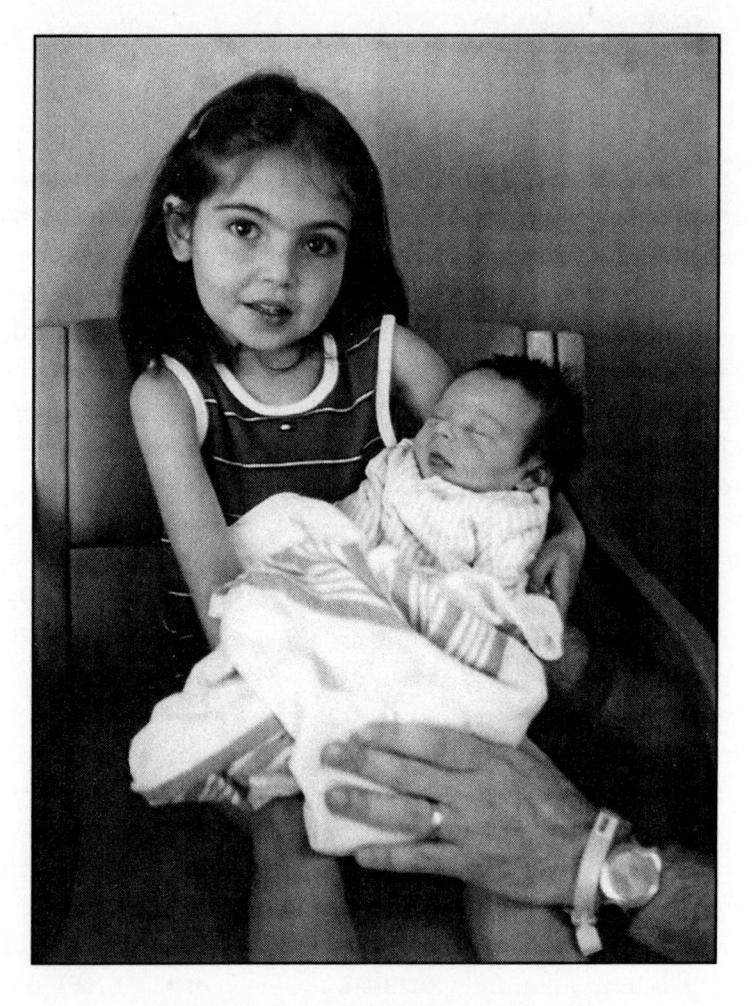

Holding baby brother Joshua, June, 2002.

she could. This was her first opportunity to be a real helper, because after Ryan's birth she was recovering from open-heart surgery and had her own physical strength to regain. So at age six, Jaclyn had a baby brother to help care for and adore, and Ryan had a sibling who is his best buddy.

Joshua was easygoing from the beginning. He went with the flow. It was nice having a new baby in the house and watching how his siblings took to him. Jaclyn helped feed Joshua bottles and then baby food, while Ryan constantly entertained him with baby and toddler toys.

For all the discussions Alan and I had about whether or not to have a third child, we simply cannot imagine life without Joshua. Jaclyn and Ryan, being three years apart, played together but also had their rivalries. She would read to him and try to teach him games, but his interests were more focused on building and tearing things apart. While she would sit still for hours playing games, doing workbooks, or making crafts, Ryan was more on the go. So when they played together, it was often initiated by me, and it was usually focused on mutually agreed upon activities—like dancing around the house, watching movies together, sledding, building snow forts, playing air hockey or darts, and making art projects. Ryan engaged in many team sports. Jaclyn played t-ball and took dance classes. However, over the years she watched and cheered for her brother in t-ball, basketball, soccer, baseball, and karate.

Joshua, on the other hand, being six years younger than Jaclyn, was intrigued by the attention she paid him. And she liked the occasional "mothering" role. It was not unusual to see Jaclyn playing with Joshua, holding his hand, reading to him, feeding him, snuggling with him, and even talking to him in a "Mommy" kind of way.

When Joshua was a baby and toddler, it was hard to juggle three children with such diverse needs. But once Joshua was walking and talking and less dependent on me, it became easier to be a mom to three children. We inevitably had an agenda, usually set by Jaclyn, for how to spend our days. The five of us were constantly on the move and loved it!

Can't this Kid Catch a Break?

I clearly remember sitting in the little room in the Pediatric Subspecialties office when Jaclyn was four weeks old, being told that she had cardiac anomalies. I recall with utmost clarity that I felt our life was changing in that very moment, never to be the same again. After meeting the surgeons for the first catheterization to determine if fixing her heart was "doable," I remember being told that her heart would be repaired by the time she was three years old. In my mind, I believed that life would be difficult until she was three, and then we would go about our lives. How wrong could I be? It had never occurred to me that cardiac problems would or could cause so many other issues.

At age two, Jaclyn followed her older cousin over the back of a couch. While her cousin made it over safely, Jaclyn fell on the hard floor, breaking her elbow. At age four, running down a slightly declined sidewalk after spending a day swimming at my mom's pool, Jaclyn tripped and landed on the same elbow and broke it again. It was explained to us that because she was so thin, breakage was a more likely event. So I worried that broken bones were going to be a part of this child's life.

At age five, the gastric surgeon entered our life when Jaclyn's gall bladder needed to be removed. As if we didn't have enough doctors and specialists in our lives, throughout the years we also took Jaclyn for second opinions. Although we always loved our heart surgeon, at one point it was recommended that we see another surgeon to see if he would treat Jaclyn's case any differently. He, in turn, referred us to a team of doctors in New York. Alan flew Jaclyn to New York City for a three-day consultation. Their recommendations were to try a new medicine to lower Jaclyn's pulmonary pressures and to put her on a waiting list at age six for a heart/lung transplant, even if she didn't need it then. That introduced a whole new can of worms to the mix. Our surgeon does not perform heart/lung transplants and had explained to us over the years that Jaclyn was not a good candidate for that surgery. She wouldn't need only a heart, but rather the combination of heart and lungs if she were to get a transplant. The problem was that survival rates for children undergoing heart/lung transplants are very, very low, so that was not going to be an option for us.

For a short time, we consulted with a behavioral psychologist about Jaclyn's eating. After a few sessions with us, he wasn't convinced Jaclyn's eating difficulties were psychological in nature. All of the medications Jaclyn took warned that a decreased appetite was a potential side effect. Together, nobody doubted that she probably had little appetite. Moreover, because she was NG-tube fed on a strict schedule as a baby, she never learned to satiate hunger.

We also consulted dieticians and nutritionists, who suggested supplementing her food with extra calories. For awhile I added butter, oil, and powdered supplements to Jaclyn's food for extra calories, but she detected the change in taste and refused to eat altogether. That defeated the purpose.

When she was seven, we took her to Milwaukee to see a team of "Eating Specialists." She was evaluated by a speech pathologist, a nutritionist, and another behavioral psychologist. The speech pathologist noted that Jaclyn seemed to favor eating crunchy foods in combination with softer, mushier foods. It was explained to us that crunchy foods get one's attention better and can sometimes be used to help clear the mouth of softer foods. We were encouraged to serve Jaclyn pretzels, chips and other crunchy items with sandwiches, chicken, and beef. At first, this seemed to help Jaclyn swallow a little better, but eventually eating got easier for her as she grew. The nutritionist suggested condiments to enhance flavors and to add calories to foods. Jaclyn didn't like the tastes of any of the high calorie foods I was encouraged to buy, but we did manage to get her to drink milkshakes and occasional high-calorie drinks, though not as often as we would have liked. While the variety of foods Jaclyn ate did increase over time, quantities were still rather small. As she got older, I was still the one who nagged and asked her to have "just a few more bites."

Because eating took a considerable amount of time for Jaclyn, the behavioral psychologist put us on a regime of eating with a timer, without punishing Jaclyn for not finishing. We were to fill her plate with a variety of textured foods (including crunchy items), but to give small servings to encourage success at finishing. We were instructed not to remind Jaclyn continuously to take bites of her food and to let her take control of her own eating. However, the behavioral psychologist had warned us that perhaps Jaclyn ate small amounts as a means of being in control of something in her life because she had little control of other aspects. By trial and error, over time we came to believe that Jaclyn simply *couldn't* eat fast. She needed to drink between bites, and chewing and holding food in her mouth for long periods of time was just the way she ate. We got used to her slow speed, and eventually as she got older, she ate a little faster.

Finally, the speech pathologist scheduled a swallow study. Jaclyn drank barium and then pictures were taken as she ate and drank. It was determined that she had enlarged tonsils that the team recommended having removed. They thought her tonsils made swallowing difficult, and that, once removed, food would go down more comfortably. However, they warned us that without tonsils, Jaclyn might have to re-learn how to swallow, possibly with a feeding tube. After our past experience with an NG-tube, that was out of the question.

A visit to an ear, nose, and throat specialist confirmed that Jaclyn's tonsils were, in fact, quite large. He too suggested removing them, with the same warning that swallowing might lead to choking for awhile for Jaclyn, necessitating a feeding tube. When we brought this recommendation to our cardiologist, he refused to allow Jaclyn to have elective surgery. First of all, any surgery for her could be dangerous. Second, there was no definitive answer as to whether removing the tonsils would indeed make eating easier for her. I was relieved that no new surgery would be forced upon us. Thankfully, my fears of another feeding tube were laid to rest.

Along the way, there have also been effects on Jaclyn's teeth from her cardiac status. Being petite meant she had a small mouth and therefore little space for permanent teeth. Subsequently, she has had many baby teeth pulled. Also, her medications affected tooth enamel, so some of her teeth discolored. It was just one more thing we dealt with.

Another medical issue Jaclyn faced was a distended stomach. When she would awaken in the morning, her stomach would be flat. She would have a dose of diuretics which made her go to the bathroom. Consequently she was thirsty and drank a lot throughout the day. By later in the afternoon, as her second dose of diuretic was due, her stomach would become somewhat distended. At night Alan used to measure the girth around her belly to see how much she was retaining fluids. Jaclyn kept a cloth tape measure on her dresser and would help Alan read the appropriate measurement. We knew what range was "normal" and when we needed to take some action. After years of this, the cardiologist trusted us enough to allow us to slightly increase Jaclyn's dosage of Lasix by one or two milliliters if her stomach was extra large on a particular day. We were taught over the years which clinical signs and symptoms could indicate problems, and we were vigilant about it. A distended stomach was one potential symptom, but we handled it appropriately.

When Jaclyn was nine years old, we began in earnest to tackle the height problem. We had asked our cardiologist about growth hormones for years. The answer was always the same: growth hormones were not recommended for children with cardiac problems because research had not yet been conducted on this population. But when Jaclyn was nine, she was still the same size as her six-year old brother, and the gap between her height and that of her friends was widening. After reading an article in a news journal about advanced developments being made in the endocrinology field, I asked our cardiologist to find out if these drugs might indeed help Jaclyn grow. It took four months to get an appointment with one of only a few pediatric endocrinologists in our area. He determined, by bone age study, that although Jaclyn was chronologically nine years old, her bone age was only six years, ten months. After weeks of consultations between the endocrinologist and our cardiologist, the two doctors decided growth hormones were worth a try—with much monitoring. This was a daily injection that we had to administer to Jaclyn. Moreover, we were told that it might take six months before we knew if the growth hormones were working. So we would be injecting our daughter with hormones for six months before we would even know if they were working—and she hated shots!

Learning to give my daughter injections was traumatic, to say the least. It was even worse than inserting the NG-tube because Jaclyn was older and more verbal about her feelings. We practiced injecting medicine from a special pen into a rubber lion. When the nurse saw we had done it properly, it was time to practice…on Jaclyn. My initial reaction, as with the NG-feeding tube, was that my husband could be in charge of this responsibility, and I wouldn't have to. But, just like the feeding tube, I was required to learn to administer the shots. Coincidentally, three days after we started the growth hormones, Alan had to be out of town for a week. I would not only have to give the shots, but I would have to do it alone that first week.

The first time I gave Jaclyn an injection, tears welled in my eyes. She was amazing through it all and never made a sound. It only took a few seconds, but because I was thinking so hard about what I was doing, it felt like it took forever! Within a month, Jaclyn grew! The hormones were working. During the previous four years, Jaclyn grew approximately one inch per year. In that first month on the growth hormones, she grew one quarter of an inch. Every month we measured her. My mom had painted a height stick covered with colorful animals when Jaclyn was a baby, and we used it over the years to measure all our children's heights. By looking at the stick, we could see how stunted Jaclyn's growth had been for years. But on the growth hormones, she was consistently growing each month. This meant she might grow three inches in one year! To us, that was remarkable.

Over time, administering the shots became less traumatic. Jaclyn got used to it and vowed that it didn't even hurt. Once in awhile we'd accidentally poke her in a vein and then she'd bruise. But otherwise, she didn't mind. When my mom learned how to give the hormone shots, Jaclyn laughed at how queasy her grandma was. It was just one more thing Jaclyn came to accept as part of her life.

Lessons Jaclyn Taught Me.

Know your child's medical history and educate yourself about it as best as you can. This is especially helpful when consulting with new doctors. Doctors often run late for appointments. Short appointments often take longer than expected. New doctors and specialists unfamiliar with Jaclyn's history often had a litany of questions to ask. I learned that if I educated myself enough to try to answer a new doctor's questions, then I could participate in the dialogue and therefore gain more information from these appointments.

I also learned how to make the most of wait time at doctor appointments. If I knew Jaclyn would need blood drawn in the lab or a chest x-ray, then I would make arrangements for the doctors to leave written orders for those tests at the reception check-in desk. When doctors were running behind, we could go to the lab or get x-rays taken first. We drove an hour to and from each cardiology appointment and usually stayed for two or three hours, while all the tests were completed. Jaclyn hated that the commute, plus the needed tests, often took half a day. She disliked missing school and other activities. So she started packing games and workbooks to take with us to appointments. We visited different doctors multiple times each year, so taking advantage of wait time, when possible, was something Jaclyn and I came to appreciate.

Hospital-Free Is a Good Way To Be

Six years passed between heart surgeries. Between the ages of three and nine, hospitals were out of our lives, except for gall bladder surgery at age six, necessitating an overnight hospital stay. Other than that, six years without a major hospitalization was much appreciated in our lives. We knew Jaclyn would need her synthetic pulmonary arteries replaced as they showed signs of wear-and-tear or became dysfunctional. We were told when she was three years old that the next surgery would probably need to be done at age six or seven, depending on her growth spurts. But in those years, there were no growth spurts. She would be nine before the fifth surgery to replace these vessels was needed. During that time, she was petite but a regular little girl…. small but mighty!

In those six years aside from her size, Jaclyn was like any other kid her age. Academically, she excelled. She read with a vengeance—to me, to Alan, to Ryan, to Joshua, and to anyone who would listen. She liked to share her thoughts about what she read too. When Joshua was a baby, my husband and I read picture books aloud at bedtime. Jaclyn soon tired of these, and when she was seven, we switched to a different bedtime ritual. Alan would read picture books to the boys, while Jaclyn and I would have Mother-Daughter reading time. We would read chapter book after chapter book—she'd read a few pages aloud to me, then I'd read to her. She began requesting to read quietly to herself after our together reading time ended. It was not unusual to

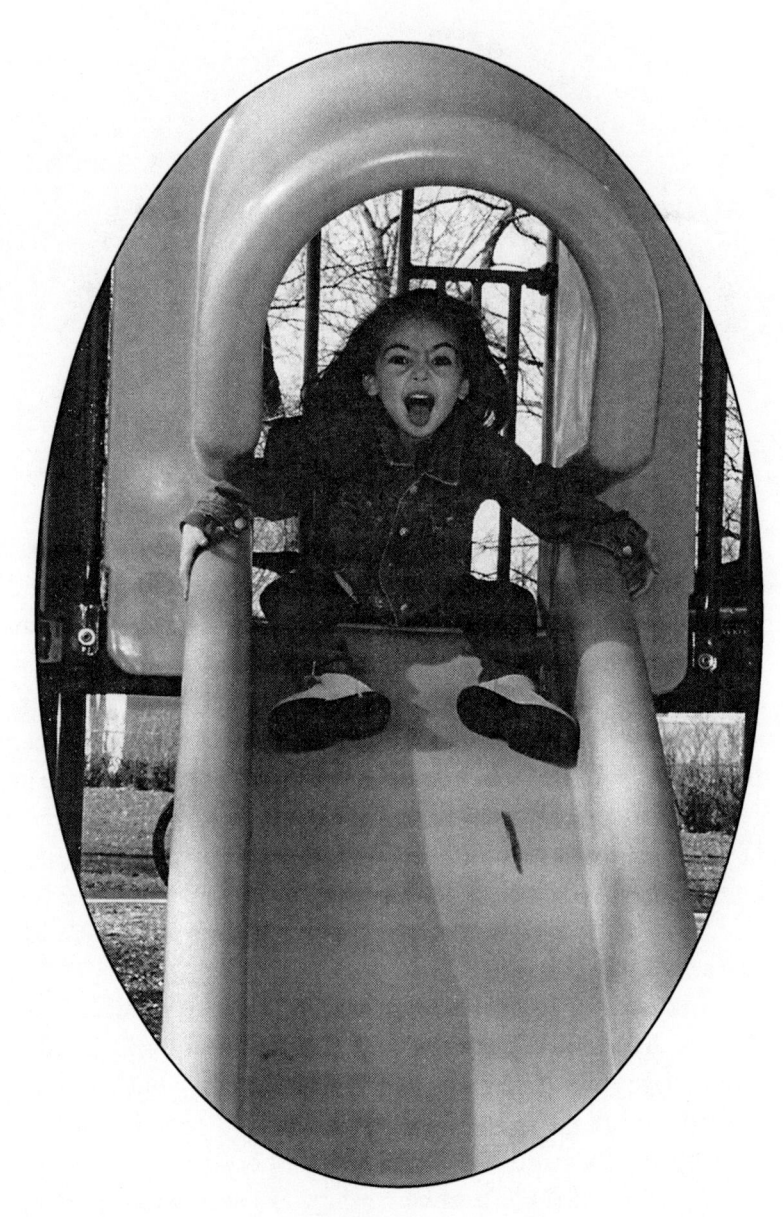

Jaclyn loved parks. Here she is acting goofy, while careening down a slide, Spring, 2002.

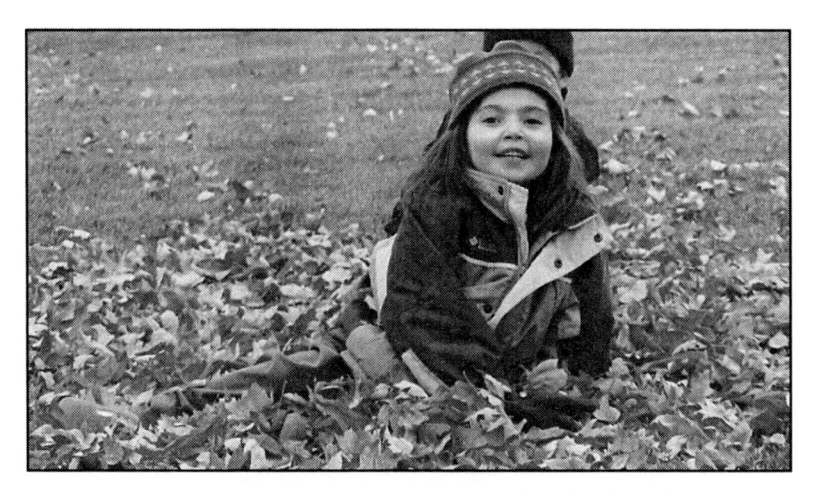

*Playing in the leaves in the backyard,
Fall, 2002.*

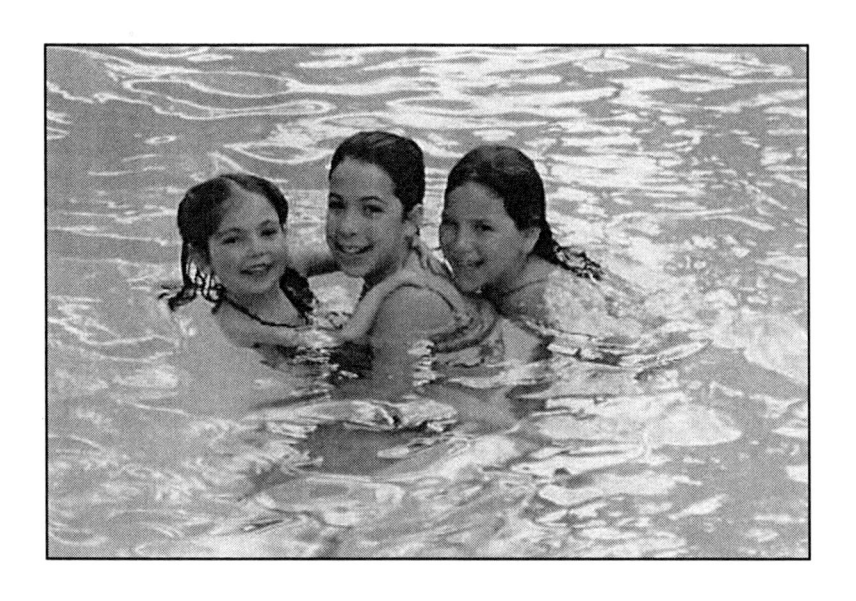

*Swimming with cousins Melissa and Megan on a trip to Florida,
December, 2002.*

remind her that it was time for lights out and to find her giggling and begging for a few more minutes. Often we'd kiss her goodnight and find her asleep with an open book on her chest, or sleeping with her hand clutching the page she was on. Jaclyn's nightstand always had a pile of books on it—school-assigned books, books we were reading together, and other books for her own quiet reading time. She poured through chapter books like they were nothing. At first with help, and then by herself, she read her way through series after series of books, as well as a variety of poetry and non-fiction books about animals too.

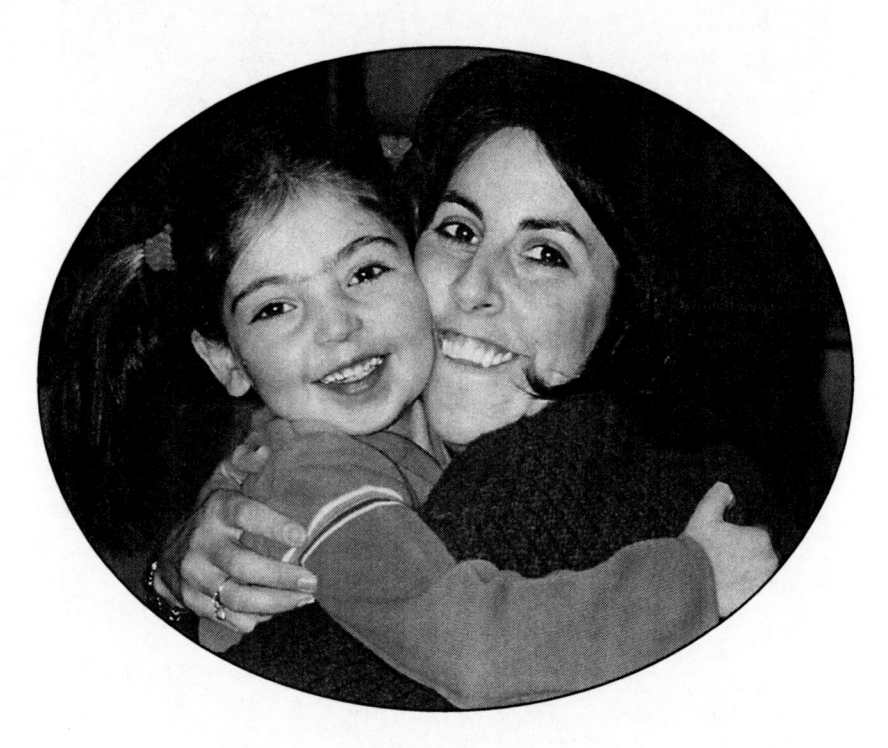

Jaclyn and Mom.

First, second, and third grade were great times for Jaclyn. The school principal encouraged students to submit jokes to be read during morning announcements. Another challenge for Jaclyn. She began to look for knock-knock books and other joke and riddle books at the library. For years, if she heard a good joke somewhere, she would scribble it down and submit it to the school office. She reveled in hearing her jokes read over the PA system. For years her friends commented that Jaclyn's jokes were read more than any other student in the school. She demonstrated that in spite of everything, humor was important.

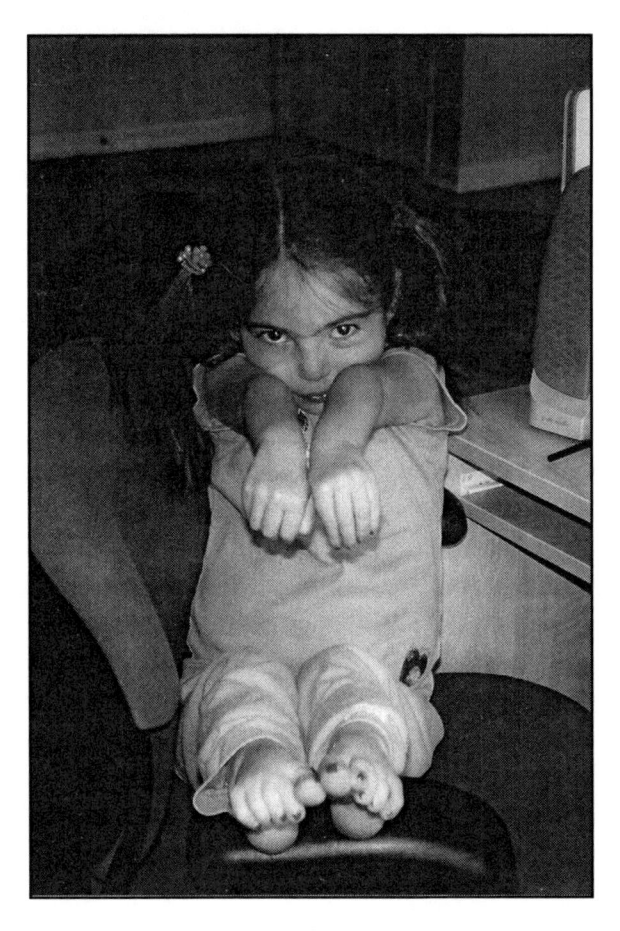

She liked to wear nail polish on her fingers and toes. But one color was not usually enough; she liked either striped polish or each nail a different color, like a rainbow.

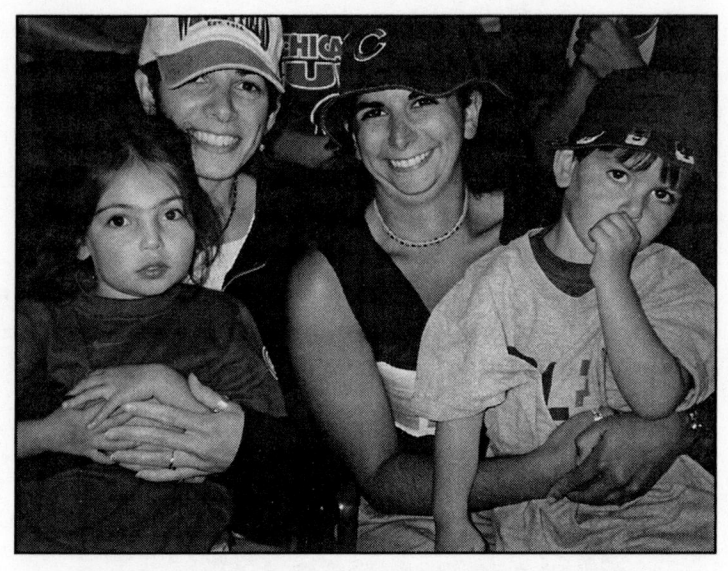

Cousin Traci and Cousin Jennifer took Jaclyn and Ryan to their first Cubs game in July, 2003.

In second grade, Jaclyn's teacher allowed students to "Putt for Perks." Receiving 100% on spelling tests would allow students to putt the shortest distance to the hole. As an avid speller, Jaclyn earned a lot of perks that year—lunch with the teacher, extra pencils, erasers, etc. I am a good speller, but Jaclyn often stumped my husband with challenge words that she could spell while he could not. Ryan and Joshua thought this was hysterical.

By third grade, Jaclyn had established herself as a diligent student and a teacher's helper. One particular teacher called Jaclyn her "go-to girl" because she was always ready to explain things to the class and answer questions. Though Jaclyn had many friends, she was always very comfortable around adults. She enjoyed helping teachers with "teacher work," often taking on the role of class secretary. She liked to hand out papers and keep track of the daily schedule. She was very organized, perhaps because her own eating and medication schedule had been so regimented for so long. Jaclyn also enjoyed eating lunch on special occasions with teachers, the school physical therapist, and the principal. There was something about the quietness of the classroom rather than the noise and busyness of the lunchroom that she found comforting.

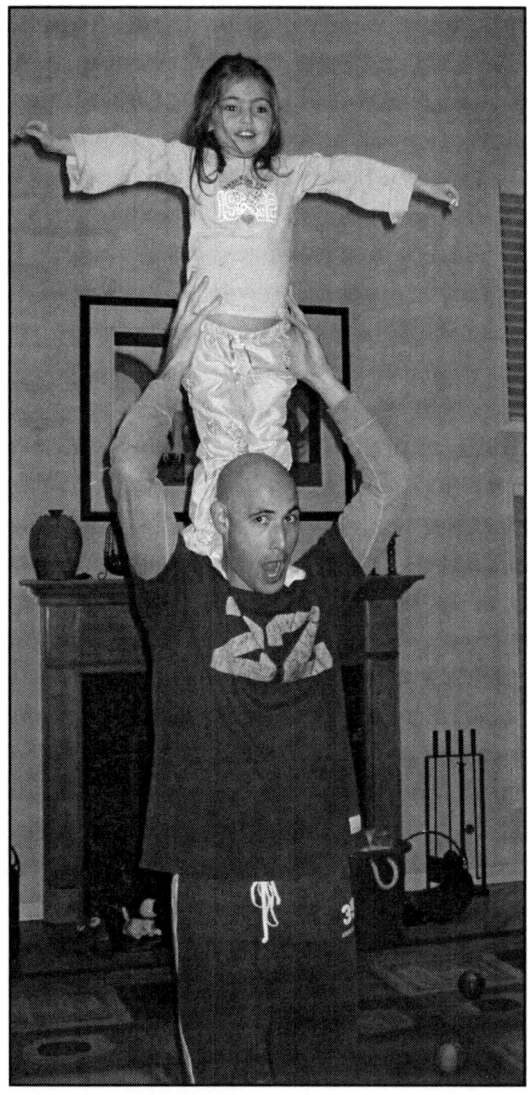

Goofing around with Uncle Danny, December, 2003.

While outside at recess, Jaclyn could often be found at the teachers' side, chatting with him/her about life outside of school, or just staying out of the shadow of boisterous children on the playground. Many days I would see her on the blacktop from my kitchen window. At first I felt badly that she didn't always play with other children. But then I realized she DID enjoy recess. She enjoyed acting grown up and talking with adults, rather than being rowdy on the playground with her peers. When her friends played Four-Square or colored the blacktop with chalk, she would join them. Other times she stayed by the teachers' side, often asking for a push on the swing. Sometimes she would walk with a friend across the school field toward our house and wave to me and her brothers. I'd often come outside for a quick hello, to see her smile, and to hear how her day was going so far. Then she'd wave and head back to recess and the rest of her school day. These brief check-ins in the middle of the day added to our special bond.

Jaclyn's desire to be around adults transferred outside of school as well. She often played with friends' moms on play dates, and wasn't intimidated to start conversations with neighbor moms and dads, or parents of her brothers' friends. She often asked if she could go across the street to "chat" with one of our neighbors. On a number of occasions I'd watch her through our window as she'd sit on their front stoop, talking through the front door to the mom and her young daughters. Her style was friendly and endearing. When she was younger and stayed by my side at get-togethers and celebrations, I tried to persuade her to play with children. But from an early age, she enjoyed the company of adults and had a maturity about her that seemed older than her years.

Physically, Jaclyn was slowly progressing during her hospital-free years. She didn't have much strength in her body or extremities, making it difficult for her to complete certain tasks. She continued to receive physical and occupational therapy through school, although I still prohibited her from missing academic class time for these appointments. Jaclyn wouldn't have it any other way! She also had private physical therapy one hour per week to supplement the school therapy. It was in these sessions that she was able to ride a bicycle, though still with training wheels. Building strength to peddle a bike took a long time to achieve, but the smile on her face when she was finally able to ride without being pushed was worth the effort. The tasks she couldn't complete on her own didn't slow her down! Jaclyn never minded asking friends to help her open certain snack containers that her fingers couldn't open. She wasn't uncomfortable requesting help to put her chair upside-down on the desk at the end of the day. And she had no qualms about needing assistance unlatching her car seat because she couldn't do it herself.

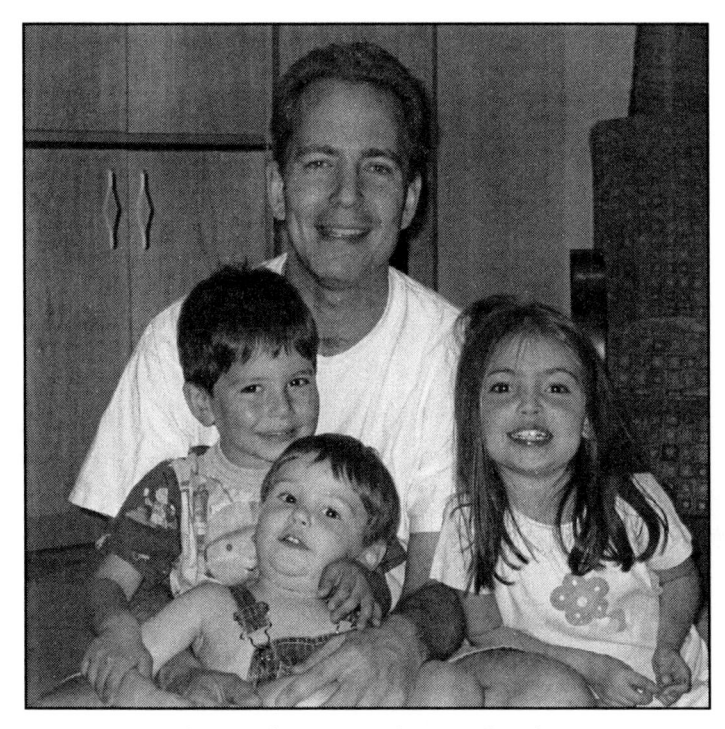

Alan with Ryan, Joshua and Jaclyn.

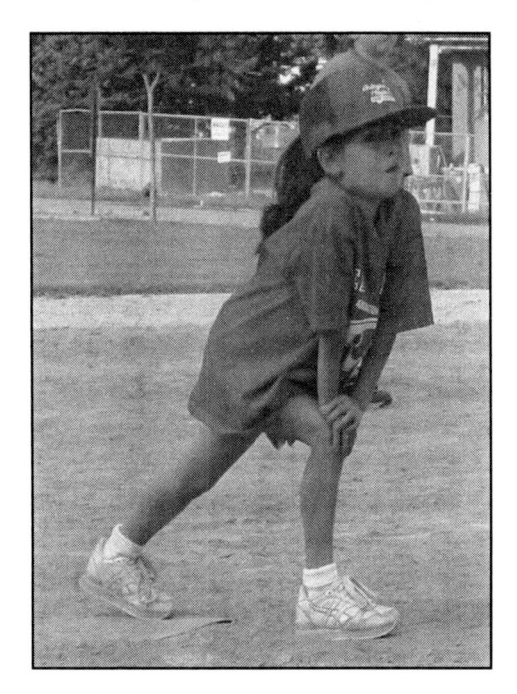

Playing on a t-ball team and waiting for a hit! (July, 2004)

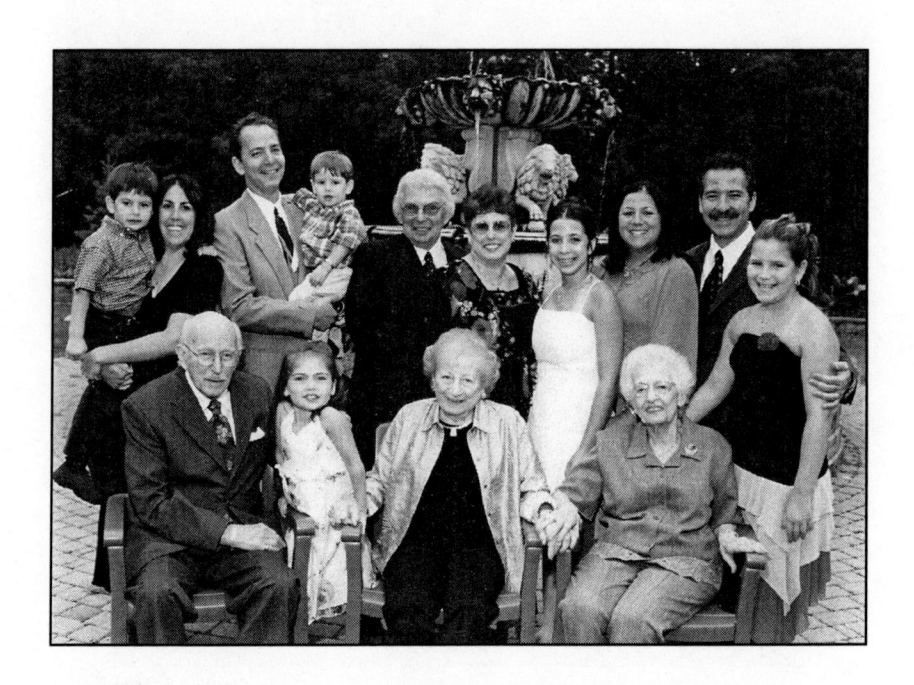

Family photo at Cousin Melissa's Bat Mitzvah, August, 2004. (Back row: Ryan, Me, Alan, Joshua, Grandpa Bob, Grandma Bobbi, Melissa, Aunt CJ, Uncle Larry, Megan; Front row: Great grandpa Al, Jaclyn, Great grandma Judy, Great grandma Irma).

Socially, there were girlfriends at our house often. Not a week went by when Jaclyn wasn't asking, "Can I have a friend over?" She had her own phone book, and she did her own inviting. She was great at booking play dates in advance. There were still a good many of her friends who didn't invite her often to their homes, but Jaclyn didn't seem to notice. I loved watching her with what were to become her best friends. Jaclyn became friends with Amber in the home daycare she attended as a toddler, and the girls maintained a close friendship. When they were younger, Amber and Jaclyn played veterinarian with a bed full of stuffed animals and a doctor's kit. As they got older, crafts and games took over their time. I'd often find them sharing a chair in front of the computer playing *Wheel of Fortune,* one of Jaclyn's favorite games.

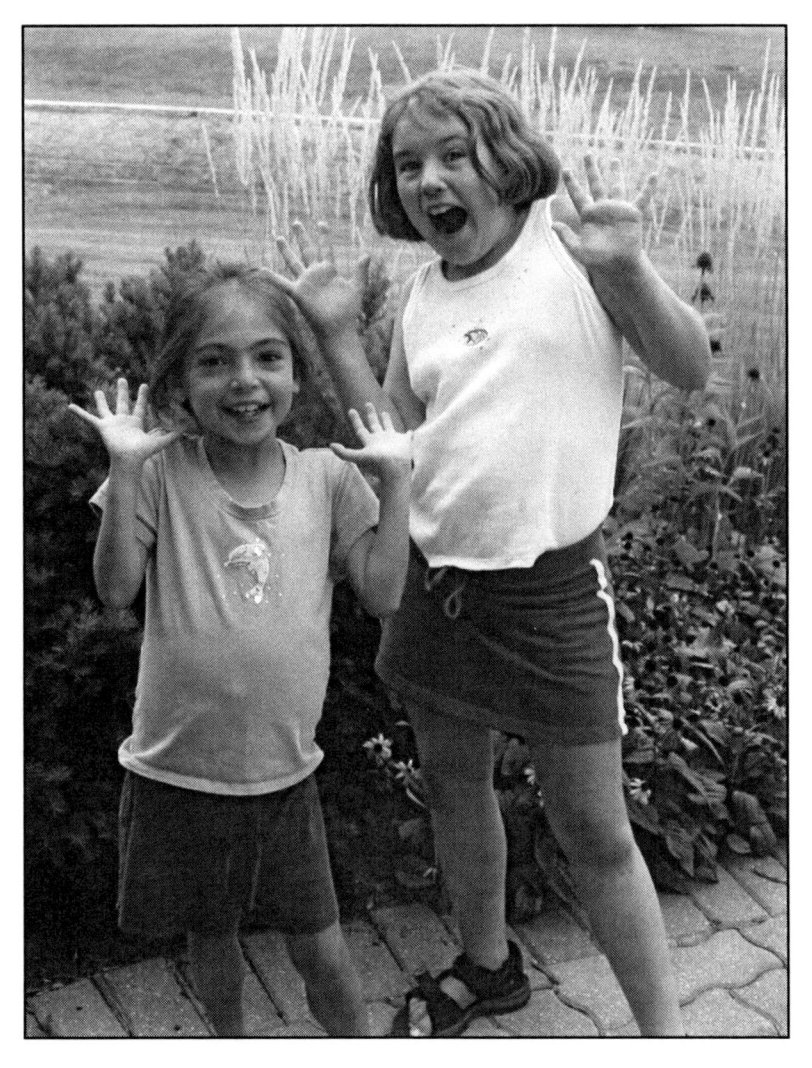

Clowning around with Amber, Summer, 2005.

In second grade, Bethany moved to our community, and the girls were together often. Jaclyn and Bethany had game marathons. A favorite was *Wordrop* where tiles are put into a board to form words across, up and down, and diagonally. When they would run out of the "good letters," I would hear them making up words or pretending uncommon letters represented more common ones. They giggled and giggled, either playing games indoors or outside under the patio umbrella. Pictures of these two smiling friends, one with long red hair and one with long dark brown hair, line a shelf in Jaclyn's room.

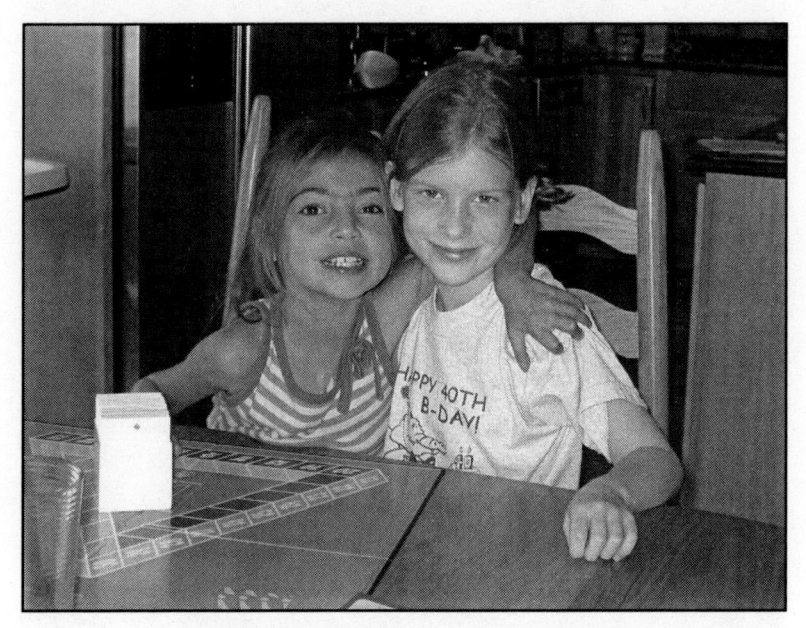

Jaclyn and Bethany, Summer, 2005.

By third grade, Jaclyn was inviting friends to sleep over, though she was not yet comfortable going to sleep at their houses. Jaclyn included most of the girls in her grade on play dates and to parties—she thought of them all as her friends.

They often played board games at the kitchen table while listening to music, or Jaclyn would ask, "Can we make a project?" and then we would lug various art supplies from the basement to their work space in the kitchen. To her friends, our house was the "craft house," as we have supplies and/or kits for just about any project imaginable. They would make sand art bottles, snap bracelets, beaded jewelry, buttons, clay animals, and often key chains out of beads. Between the games I had saved from my own childhood and the ones we bought for our strategically craving child, we have them all! The sight of little girls blaring music while playing games brought a smile to my face.

During those hospital-free days, I also was one of Jaclyn's friends. We enjoyed being with each other, while Ryan and Joshua busied themselves with Legos, building, and racing cars. We played games at all times of the day and night. We could sneak in a quick game of *Racko* or *Yahtzee* before school. We could play *Hangman* while making dinner. *Mad Libs* were another favorite, as Jaclyn often asked us for nouns, adjectives or whatever part of speech the directions called for. Other times she filled in the blanks by herself, then read the stories back and laughed at the absurdity of them. I loved that she loved so many things I did. I relished that she enjoyed music and that she danced around the family room. Parents aren't supposed to say their children are their friends, but my children are and I'm not ashamed of that.

Music was a big part of Jaclyn's life. As a baby and toddler, she listened to music tapes in the car or on a little tape recorder my mom bought for her first hospital stay. Then she moved on to children's music videos and played with musical instruments. As she got older, she enjoyed Broadway musicals on DVD and especially loved going to musical theatre in downtown Chicago. My mom and I indulged Jaclyn, Ryan and Joshua with tickets to many musicals over the years. She loved the live performances of *The Sound of Music, Peter Pan, Beauty and the Beast, The Lion King,* and especially *Wicked*. The joke in our family was that whenever we'd be heading somewhere in the car, we could always count on Jaclyn to select a bunch of CDs for the ride.

Music played all the time at our house, inside and outside. Jaclyn choreographed numbers so she and her brothers could "put on shows" for us. It was hysterical. The funniest number was "So Long, Farewell" from *The Sound of Music* that Jaclyn choreographed with her brothers. Jaclyn, Ryan, and then Joshua would dance the steps the way Jaclyn interpreted them from watching the movie numerous times. All three of them loved to perform! They liked the applause.

Jaclyn began taking piano lessons when she was eight. Teachers recommended waiting until her hands were bigger before beginning lessons, but because we assumed she would always be petite, we pushed forward and found a teacher. Jaclyn caught on immediately and enjoyed the piano immensely.

During those hospital-free years, we continued to have regular doctor appointments and faced occasional hurdles. Jaclyn received at least five different medications daily for many of those years, each requiring more than one dose per day. Medicine was simply part of life. At some point, it was also determined that supplemental oxygen could help her when she slept. Her oxygen levels were still not "normal," but rather in the lower 90s. When asleep, her levels often dipped into the 80s. We had gotten rid of the oximeter and the Kangaroo feeding pump years earlier, but we were now the proud owners of an oxygen concentrator. As part of her bedtime ritual, Jaclyn would pull her hair into a ponytail and adjust the oxygen cannula into her nose. When she was asleep, we would turn on the machine. Because the oxygen was only recommended, Jaclyn often had sleepovers at my mom's house without it. When we travelled, we always arranged for oxygen to be installed in our hotel room for the duration of our stay. It was another one of those things Jaclyn never complained about, but rather just accepted as part of her life.

Jaclyn also made great strides in her eating during the years. As a young child she struggled with texture issues as well as quantity issues, and eating was painstakingly slow for her. The variety of foods she consumed was minimal. But during the hospital-free years, Jaclyn developed a new interest in tastes and foods. It was amazing that the same child who had been tube-fed, and who had terrible texture issues when she ate at all, could grow up to count barbeque ribs, steak, and popcorn as her favorites. The texture issues had finally faded. The quantity of foods she ate was still quite small, so we resorted to multiple snacks throughout the day to supplement her. I would push for high-calorie snacks, such as peanut butter on apple slices, or a bowl of nuts, or one of Jaclyn's favorites—peanut butter on Bugle chips. Often she would opt for a bowl of Goldfish crackers at 2 ½ calories per cracker. The twenty crackers she would consume weren't nearly the amount of calories I would have liked her to have, but at least she was eating something.

Jaclyn went through a phase where all she ate for breakfast was ice cream. Rather than making a big deal of this, we referred to ice cream as "dairy" (making it sound somewhat healthy) and let it go. In my mind, this particular "dairy" constituted a high-caloric meal. Months later she wanted bacon every morning for breakfast. I hated frying it daily, but it was high in calories, and she liked it, so fry I did.

Arguing with Jaclyn about what to eat, how much to eat, how often to eat, and how slowly she was eating consumed an overabundance of time and patience over the years. When she was younger, I was crazed about her caloric intake because she was small and her hard-working heart was still burning a lot of her calories. I knew exactly how much went into her body each day. As she got older, I eased up a little, though I still felt pressure about getting more calories into her if I could. I'd walk up and down grocery store aisles looking for granola bars, yogurts and other snacks with high numbers of calories. One shelf in the panty was designated the "Jaclyn shelf" because it contained high calorie foods that the rest of our family members didn't need.

For many years we put hospital life behind us. We had three kids. We travelled a lot. We went to Los Angeles, Disney World, Minneapolis, Cincinnati, San Diego, Dallas, Port St. Lucie-Florida, Seattle, Portland, Phoenix, West Palm Beach, Cleveland, and the Wisconsin Dells. We went on special outings. Jaclyn often served as our event planner. During spring, winter, and summer vacations, and on days off of school, she would be the first to come up with potential activities to fill our days—the public pool, the zoo, the many museums in Chicago, the nearby arcade, miniature golfing, bowling, movies, painting ceramics, favorite restaurants for breakfast or lunch, or just play dates at home with friends. She would be the one to ask if we could get together with other families on the weekends.

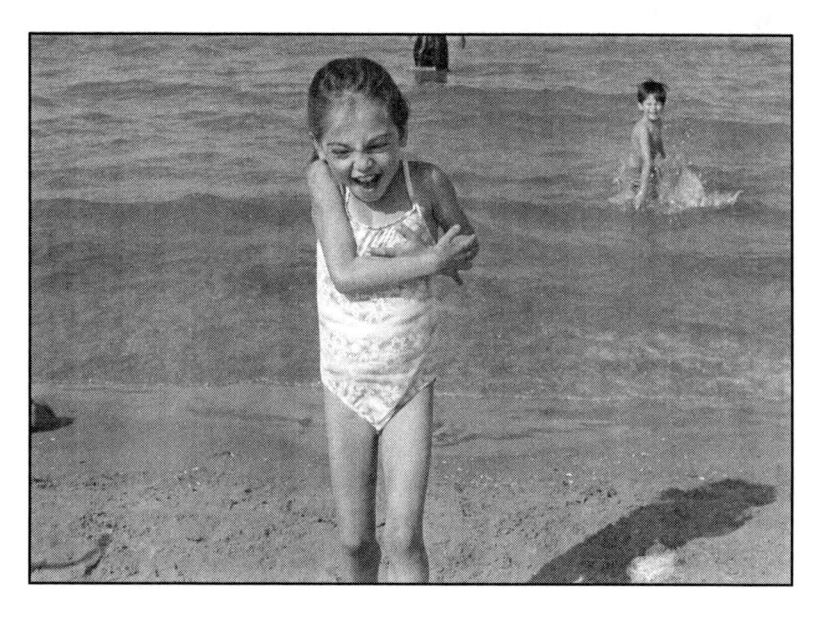

"It's freezing!" (at the beach during Summer, 2005).

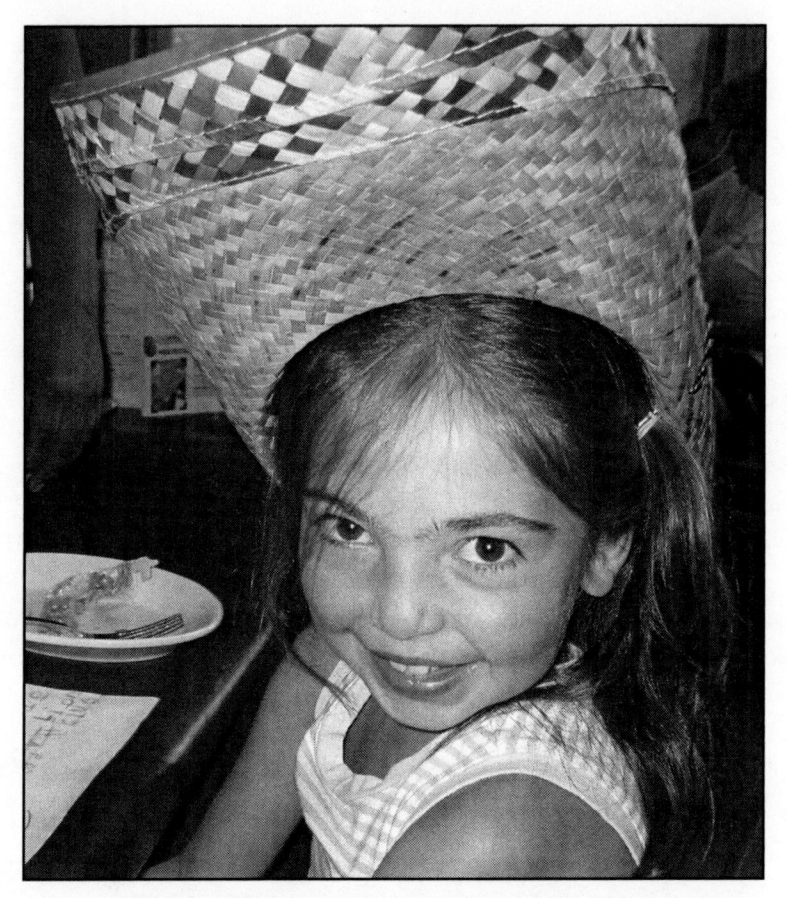

At a Mexican restaurant to celebrate a birthday.

  Jaclyn was constantly challenging herself with extra activities as well, such as search and find puzzles, word games, and Sudoko. She filled her days reading the sports page and the weather section of the *Chicago Tribune*, making up dance steps to go with songs she knew, reading books, doing puzzles, baking and helping me make dinner, coloring the driveway with chalk drawings, making crafts, taking great effort to make elaborate birthday cards for family and friends, and, always playing games. In the spring and summer months, Jaclyn and her brothers manned a lemonade stand in our backyard by the Little League field. On hot days, their pink lemonade stand did very well. She made a poster announcing that all money collected would be donated to the Heart Institute for Children, a charity from our surgeon's hospital.

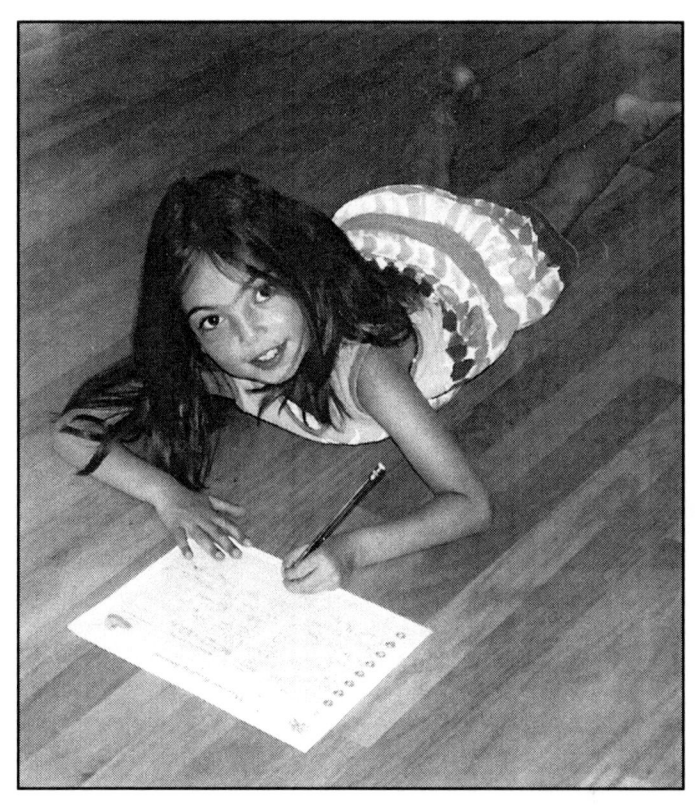

Jaclyn earned free books by participating in a summer reading program, (July, 2005).

Jaclyn also entered drawing and writing contests. One year she won a newspaper contest telling why she wanted someone else's "junk." She collected key chains, and with my assistance, had written a short essay as to why she wanted someone else's old collection to add to her own. Her entry won. The newspaper printed it, and she was ecstatic. She never passed up the chance to enter a contest for children her age. She had boundless energy. She was active, cheerful and exuberant—a far cry from what the doctors always expected to see from what her medical chart read.

Jaclyn's days were busy entertaining herself, playing with her brothers or with girlfriends, and making an impression on everyone she met. Her friends' parents often told us how polite Jaclyn was at their homes or how her personality seemed older than her years.

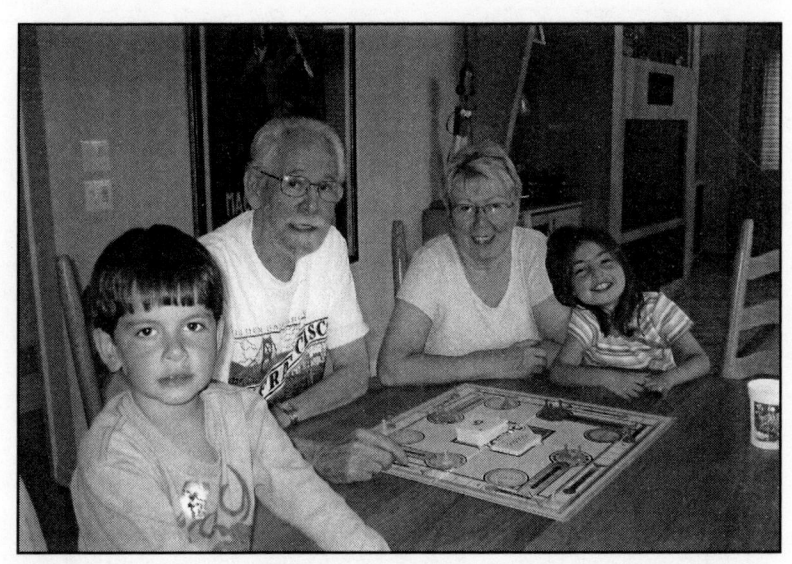

Ryan, Grandpa George, Grandma Nancy and Jaclyn playing "Sorry."

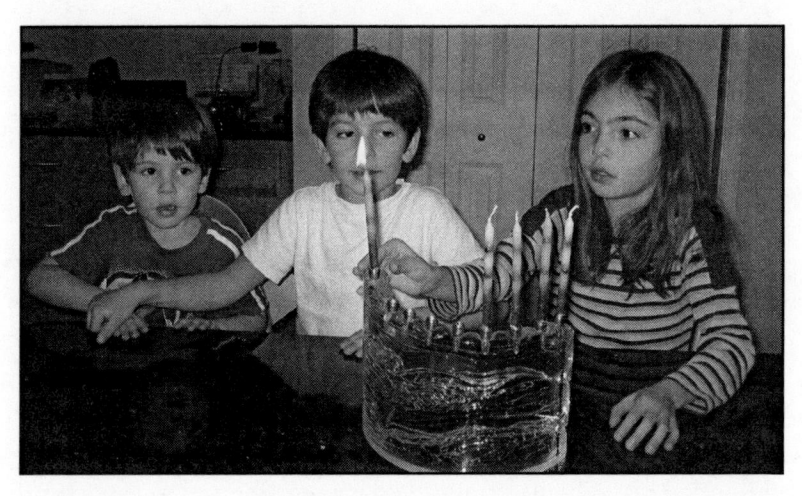

Joshua, Ryan and Jaclyn lighting the Hanukkah menorah, December, 2005.

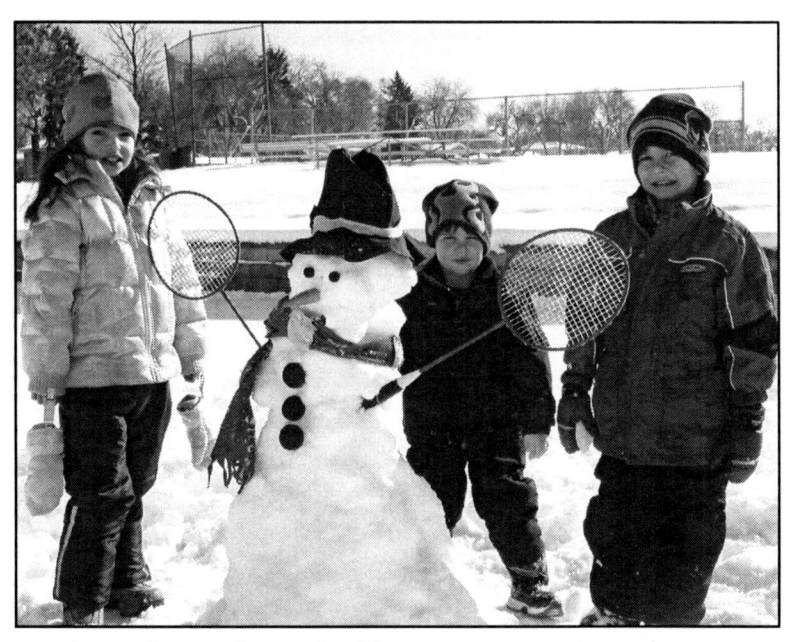

Jaclyn, Joshua and Ryan building a snowman, December, 2005.

During this time, Jaclyn also developed an even better sense of self-esteem. She was short and somewhat weak, but never shy. School was her turf, and she used to strut through those halls with an air about her. Outside of school, she took occasional dance classes, was a Girl Scout, took piano lessons, and began Hebrew school.

We continued private PT one day each week, separate from school. Her repertoire of games grew to now include computer games, X-box games and darts. She blew bubbles and entertained the younger neighborhood girls. Outside on nice days, our driveway was often covered with beautiful colored chalk drawings and the occasional *Hangman* game.

Our family developed and maintained many traditions during these years too. From an early age, Jaclyn and I made crafts because we were home a lot and it was fun. As the years went on, we started to combine Jaclyn's May birthday with Mother's Day and had one big celebration. All three kids and I made crafts to give to others. We didn't just give these gifts to the mothers in attendance but rather to all the ladies, because, according to Jaclyn, "that would make it fair." Each year we made close to twenty such gifts. One year our gifts were personalized sun visors. Another year we made frames decorated with pom-poms, sequins and glitter. One time we gave out hand-painted magnets. We also painted ceramic planters and trays. We would start weeks before Mother's Day just to finish all our gifts in time. One year for Father's Day we made tie-dye shirts for all the men in the extended family. Our biggest undertaking was the year we made hand-made calendars as Hanukkah gifts. Each page contained photographs of my three kids, put together like a scrapbook. Together, we cut, glued, measured and personalized each month in these calendars. Every calendar we made was unique. We gave them to grandparents, great-grandparents and some aunts/uncles and cousins too.

We started and maintained other family traditions as well. For years, Alan has made chocolate chip banana pancakes for Sunday breakfast. Friday Night Movie Night took place on weekends when we didn't have other activities or events. We would put on our pajamas, snuggle with sleeping bags, stuffed animals and blankets, eat lots of popcorn, and watch a movie together. On weeknights, Jaclyn would often ask, "Can I watch the *Final Puzzle*?" She tried to catch *Wheel of Fortune* on television after dinner, but often we would still be eating, so she'd try to at least watch the last puzzle of the night. I'd often abandon washing dinner dishes and plop on the couch to try to solve the final puzzle with her. We usually got it. And when Alan was out of town, the kids traditionally slept in my bed with me, or Ryan and Joshua would sleep in Jaclyn's room with her, on the floor next to her bed with their many stuffed animals. Despite occasional discussions of her heart or her petite size, Jaclyn did not think of herself as "sick." The doctors never put any restrictions on her, and she was, instead, encouraged to do whatever she felt able to do. What she couldn't do, she easily replaced with what she could. Because of her outgoing personality and that wonderful smile, people often could not believe she had cardiac problems. Our family, and especially Jaclyn, did not let her heart condition dictate or deter us from doing "normal" things.

Lessons Jaclyn Taught Me.
I never really thought about the cliché that says to "live life to its fullest," but I guess that describes how we lived. Fill your time. Have fun. Establish and maintain family traditions. Jaclyn taught us that a medical condition doesn't have to dictate life. She didn't let it consume her, and we're so very grateful for that lesson.

Being Different

Other than Jaclyn being smaller than her peers, nobody could ever tell that anything was out of the ordinary. However, the older she got, the more we noticed what she could not, or did not, do compared to her friends. While most kids loved to play outdoors, Jaclyn didn't. Though repaired, her heart would never be "normal." Her body would always work hard, making her hot, especially during the summer. "Ozone alert days" were problematic for Jaclyn, as it was dangerous for her to be in the heat when breathing was more difficult. When Jaclyn was about three years old, I would fill my whirlpool bathtub on hot summer days, dress her in a bathing suit, and let her play in the air-conditioned bathroom instead of outside in a pool. When Ryan and Joshua were old enough, all three of them would wear bathing suits and enjoy the fun of the tub. I would sit on the bathroom floor and read a magazine while they splashed and laughed. As she got older, her friends spent countless hours outside. But Jaclyn enjoyed being inside in air conditioning. She always found things to do, and she either didn't notice or simply didn't care that others were outside all the time without her.

Jaclyn was always one of the smallest children in her class. In second grade, at the age of seven, Jaclyn and Ryan, age four, were actually very close in height. This presented some unique experiences; Jaclyn despised when strangers talked to her as if she were younger. There's a high-pitch tone of voice people use when talking to young children. Jaclyn was insulted; after all she was not a baby, she was just small for her age.

As she got older, clothes became a problem because of her size. At age nine, she was still wearing size 6 pants and size 7 shirts. Her shoes were a child's size 11 or 12. There were few styles that were age-appropriate in the sizes she needed. We did a lot of hunting for older-looking clothes that actually fit. Because of weakness in her hands, Jaclyn couldn't snap or button pants. She wore stretch leggings and shorts with elastic or dresses. Shopping for clothes was a challenge, but we met it.

School presented additional challenges because of Jaclyn's height. Overall, we were fortunate to be in a small school district where virtually every family knew every other family. The kids had some knowledge of Jaclyn's medical history and needs, simply because she missed a good amount of school due to illness, surgery and other procedures. For many years Jaclyn looked the size of Ryan's classmates, and her own peers began to tower over her. There were many times she would complain about being called "shrimp" or other derogatory terms. We encouraged her to express herself the best she could and to tell kids, "It hurts my feelings when you call me names." It really upset her when kids would pick her up just to show how strong they were, or when they would measure the top of her head to their chests to show how much taller they were. That was hard for us as parents because we knew her self-esteem was tied to this, and we also knew it would probably never end.

At home we spent a lot of time talking about people being different. I hope these discussions instilled a tolerance for diversity in all of my children, in part because the five of us lived through some of the insensitivities that Jaclyn endured.

Being small was only one difference among many that Jaclyn lived with. Because of a lack of strength and endurance, certain activities that her friends participated in were not of interest to her. Bicycle riding was not something she could do, except with training wheels and only for very short distances. At a certain point, she became conscious of having training wheels when her peers did not, and that was the end of her bike-riding. We had put off teaching Ryan to ride a two-wheeler as long as we could for fear of how it would make Jaclyn feel to see her younger brother mastering a skill she could not.

Neither Alan nor I pushed the subject of bike-riding with Jaclyn. We realized it was somewhat embarrassing for her. As soon as Ryan's training wheels came off, Jaclyn had a renewed desire to conquer the same feat. Competition was a good motivator, but bike-riding without training wheels continued to evade her abilities.

Soccer was a popular sport that her friends participated in, beginning in kindergarten. Jaclyn didn't like physical games. Although she had no physical limitations placed upon her, she simply could not run as fast or as far as her friends, or jump for any significant length of time. Swimming became a big issue by second and third grade when her friends began excelling in lessons and joined swim teams. I could only imagine how it must have felt for almost every child to be on a soccer team or a swim team while she was not. Jaclyn not only missed out on the activities, but on the socializing that occurred at those events as well. When she was invited to swimming parties, either Alan or I had to get in the water with her, highlighting her inabilities more.

Jaclyn realized early on that she wasn't as good at physical things and subsequently turned to other activities. It's not that we didn't try sports, but rather that she wasn't comfortable playing many of them. She played t-ball in pre-school, but when t-ball became softball at older ages, she wasn't able to play. Our physical therapist recommended Buddy Baseball, a league in which children with disabilities were paired with able-bodied "buddies" to help them field, bat, and run bases. Many of the children on Jaclyn's team were nonverbal or physically impaired. Jaclyn played one season but had no interest in continuing.

Despite season after season of both public and private swimming lessons, swimming was still very difficult for her. But she liked it. During the summer, Jaclyn loved to go to the park district pool, especially because many of her friends were there. However, she could not go into the deep end of the pool by herself because she was not a strong enough swimmer, and it was hard to find friends who were willing to stay in shallow water with her. Her friends might play with her at the shallow end of the pool for a while, but eventually they wanted to jump off the diving board or swim in deeper water. Jaclyn would be quite disappointed when they would abandon her for the diving boards. This was heartbreaking to watch.

As she got older, Jaclyn had the idea to bring a ball to the pool.

This way she could stand outside of the pool and throw the ball to her friends in deeper water. She was learning how to adapt her play in order to continue interacting with friends.

While playing many sports was not a reality, Jaclyn developed a love of watching sports instead. From an early age she became an ardent Cubs fan. By the time she was eight, she was reading the morning sports section to see if her team had won the night before. She checked the standings, who the next opponent was, and who the starting pitcher would be. She knew every player's name, understood the rules, and watched games whenever she could. The five of us went to several Cubs games throughout the years, and my cousins also indulged Jaclyn and Ryan with Cubs tickets. In the off-season, the Cubs train in Arizona. In March, 2005, we took a trip to Phoenix and attended a Spring Training game. We had heard that Cubs players often sign autographs as they leave the stadium. Even though it meant missing part of the game, Jaclyn insisted on waiting to get an autograph, with hundreds of other fans. She was terribly disappointed to come home empty-handed.

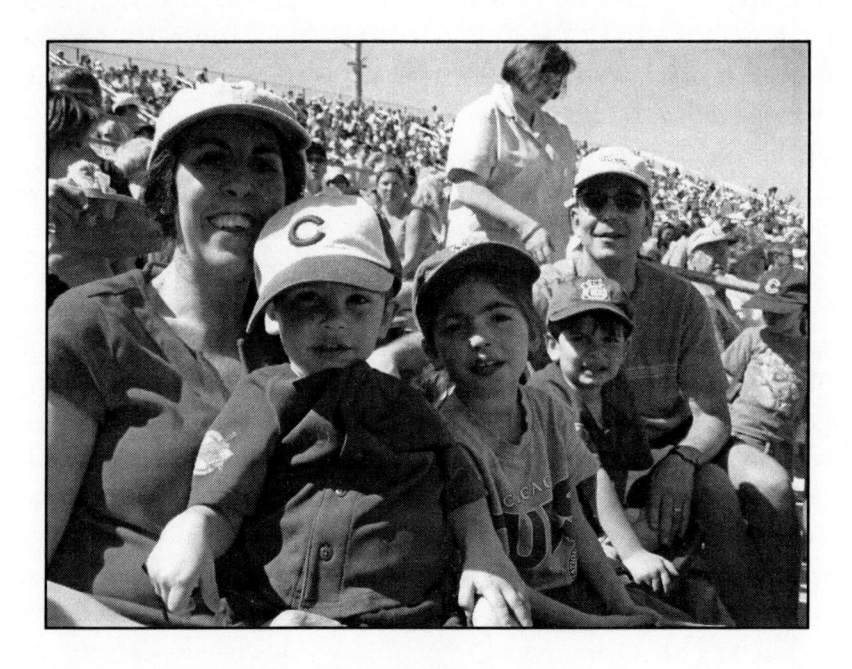

We took a trip to Phoenix in March, 2005 to see the Cubs in Spring Training.

During fall and winter, Jaclyn cheered for the Bears and the University of Illinois basketball team. Our family enjoys playing and watching sports, and Jaclyn was a regular sports fanatic. She knew all the games and the rules even though most of her girlfriends were not interested.

Since Jaclyn was scared of being trampled over on a soccer field and couldn't balance well enough for roller skating or skate boarding, she chose indoor endeavors to master instead. She was already playing board games at a young age because that was something she excelled in. They continued to be a fascination of Jaclyn's and something she was truly successful at. By the age of five and six, she was replacing the junior version of games with the adult versions. As she got older, it would not be unusual for her to use all seven of her *Scrabble* tiles to form a word; she'd laugh as she'd add the fifty-point bonus to her score. She thrived on trivia games and games that required strategy, not just luck. *Mastermind, Clue, Outburst, Battleship, Othello,* and *Trivial Pursuit* were favorites of hers, as were word games of any kind *(Boggle, Hangman, Wheel of Fortune, Upwords, Wordrop, Smart Mouth and Mad Libs).* When she could coerce someone to play for hours on end, *Monopoly* and *Life* were top choices. Years ago, when she would invite friends over, they would play games. But some of her peers were playing games that Jaclyn had outgrown, so she was different in that way too.

Taking medicine made Jaclyn different because she was required to take so many throughout the day and night. When friends came over after school, Jaclyn quickly gulped two syringes of liquid medicine and then they would go on their merry way. But by the time she began third grade, I noticed some of her friends' stares. Jaclyn didn't seem to care if her friends saw her take medicine; it was simply part of her day. I was the one who decided this no longer needed to be a public affair. To make it more private, Jaclyn would take her medicine while her friends washed their hands or used the bathroom.

If she went to a friend's house instead of coming home, we handled medicine differently. When she was younger, I used to bring her home for medicine and would then drive her to a friend's house. As she got older, Jaclyn wanted to be able to walk or ride home with a friend. It was important that she be like the other kids in as many ways as possible. In those cases, I made arrangements to drop the medicine off at her friends' houses during the day.

Over the years Alan, as well as some of Jaclyn's doctors and surgeons, commented to me about my attention to aesthetics. There were *not* a lot of things I could control regarding Jaclyn's health status, but I could at least ask about making scars less conspicuous, if possible. I was sensitive to the number of scars being added to my daughter's chest and body. As a child, I had a quarter-size, brown birthmark on my stomach. I hated it and the older I got, the more aware I became of it. I remember having to change into a high school gym uniform in front of everyone in the locker room. Horrifying! I used to stand as close to the inside of my locker as possible while changing clothes so nobody could see my stomach. When I was seventeen, my mother and I agreed that it was time to have the birthmark removed.

I was the one who feared insensitive comments about Jaclyn's marks and scars. And she was covered with them! She had a long incision down the middle of her chest, one under each arm that wrapped toward her back, numerous chest tube holes, a scar from her gall bladder surgery, and another scar in front of her armpit from the pacemaker she got at age nine. She also had additional scars around her bikini line from triple lumen IVs and multiple cardiac catheterizations. Jaclyn wasn't worried about scars. I was, because of my own memories of how mean other children could be. While I realized the surgeons had to do what they did, I requested that they minimize scars when they could, and they obliged by opening her skin in places where previous scars already existed.

One day, at age three, Jaclyn was drying off from a bath. She was standing naked in front of her full-length mirror and yelled out, "Mommy, come here. There's something wrong!" I began to run. She said, "Mommy, I have holes in my body!" I started to panic. I had imagined having a conversation with her someday about her body—how it looked, that her scars were really unimportant, and that beauty was from within, etc. But at that moment, I wasn't ready for that talk. I thought, *She's only three. It can't be time yet!* My heart raced faster as I reached her room. There she was, looking at her chest in the mirror, pointing to her nipples, saying, "Look! Something's wrong! I have owies!" I burst into laughter. The child was totally naked, she had multiple scars, and she was pointing to her nipples, asking what they were. She obviously had a good sense of herself, perhaps because she knew no other body but her own.

Alan and I have spoken about how the teen years could be especially hard for Jaclyn, as self-esteem and boys become more of an issue. In my mind I will be ready to have that conversation with her. Or perhaps she will never ask. The day Jaclyn was curious about nipples made me aware that perhaps her scars are just simply a part of her body that she is used to. She never saw herself without those scars. This was simply the way she looked.

One more difference we dealt with regarding Jaclyn and her peers had to do with independence. Jaclyn was always more dependent on us than her friends were on their parents. At almost age ten, I became more aware of encouraging her independence. But at the same time, this notion scared me. Jaclyn noticed her friends riding their bikes in the neighborhood or playing outside without parents present. She was always the first to ask where the parents were. I explained that many parents allow their children to be outside unsupervised. Jaclyn was not comfortable with that idea because she was always used to being in the presence of adults.

I also lived with a paranoid fear of leaving her alone. She was only home alone a few times by herself, for perhaps ten minutes at the most. The school is in our backyard so if she was home sick and I had to run to pick up her brothers, she could see me from the window the whole time I was gone. But I had these perhaps ridiculous fears about what could happen to her while alone. I conjured up all kinds of imaginary scenes in my head, and none were very comforting. I worried that she could have a cardiac problem in my absence. Or that if she were injured and needed to call 911, no adult would be around to explain her medical condition or her medications to paramedics. I also had an irrational fear that she could be kidnapped and miss dosages of medicines. Overprotective? Absolutely. Paranoid? Certainly. But her medical situation was precarious enough to put these thoughts in my head. And since I was responsible for her, I did take extra precautions to keep Jaclyn safe. If I stifled her independence a bit, I justified it as a small price to pay for knowing her whereabouts and that she was all right.

Friends and relatives used to call me overprotective of my children, especially Jaclyn. But until others walked in my shoes and knew all that we had been through with this child, and all we lived with, I discounted their hints about allowing my children less motherly oversight. I never hovered over Jaclyn. She went to friends' houses and did regular things with them. But I always knew where she was, and when she was in my house, I was there too. She came with me when I went out. Of course, there were times I would have liked the alone time to go out without children, but Jaclyn usually finagled her way into joining me on even mundane errands. "Can I come? Can I come?" she'd implore. I'd smile watching her pick the produce at the grocery store or listen to her order her favorites from the deli counter. She always got it right—"a half pound of Sara Lee Honey Turkey, cut-thin, please" or "I'd like one quarter of a pound of kosher beef bologna." She also loved to pick out gifts for others, often asking, "Isn't this adorable?" as she'd pull something from a store rack. Jaclyn liked to be with me, and I liked having her with me.

Lessons Jaclyn Taught Me.

Be comfortable with yourself. Let people know if they hurt your feelings, because keeping it to yourself won't change the situation. If you tell them, then at least you know that YOU'VE done all you can do to make it better. There's nothing you can do if they don't change, but it's important to know that you have tried.

Existing on the Fringe

As I have shared, physical activity and general boisterous outdoor play were areas Jaclyn often avoided. Being away from the activities that other children and families participated in made both Jaclyn and our family feel excluded in many ways over the years.

There is a lot of socializing that occurs at team sport practices and games. And when neighbors congregate outside while their kids ride bikes or roughhouse, there is a lot of social interaction occurring as well. Because Jaclyn avoided these activities, and because she played indoors more than outdoors, it was not until Ryan was old enough to participate in sports and other activities that we even realized how much we had been missing.

As Jaclyn aged, this sense of our family living on the fringe continued. I remember sitting with other parents outside a waiting room during Jaclyn's forty-five minute dance class. This was one of the first times I had the opportunity to just sit and talk with other adults. It was from these outings that I learned what was happening in school, or what other girls were up to, or the intricacies of little girls' lives. But this feeling was a double-edged sword. While I was finally privy to "Mom Talk," I was also becoming aware of all the activities my child had been left out of. I heard about other children's birthday parties and sleepovers that Jaclyn hadn't been invited to. It never had occurred to me that second graders were sleeping at each other's houses yet. It broke my heart to learn that they had been doing it for some time, and my daughter had never been invited.

    I have talked to many friends about these feelings. Some chalk it up to people not wanting to invite Jaclyn because they never knew what her limitations were. She had none. I wish people had just *asked* if Jaclyn could or couldn't do something before they discounted her. It was hurtful to be left out. It was painful for Jaclyn, and it was hard for us, as her parents to watch. Because of all our time together, Jaclyn and I were friends. Even when she was a toddler, we enjoyed being together. It hurt me to know that others were not getting to know this funny, smart, silly, competitive, caring child the way I was able to know her.

    We, as a family, have always gone out of our way to invite kids to our house. From the time Jaclyn began pre-school, I made it a point to invite friends to our house for her to play with. She had been away from children a lot her first few years because of germs, and I felt it was important for her to have many opportunities for peer play. So I began to invite her classmates over. The flip side to this was that I could learn more about what toddlers and then little girls were "supposed" to be doing at particular ages by watching them. Then I could work with Jaclyn on those endeavors. It was a win-win situation.

    As Jaclyn got older, she began filling her own calendar with play dates. She invited different friends over a few times each week. But **she did** not get invited to others' houses nearly as often as others came to our home. I didn't mind the lack of reciprocity, at least not at first. After awhile, Jaclyn began to ask why particular friends seldom asked her to come over to play.

    The same was true for birthday parties. Jaclyn consistently invited the same fourteen girls to her birthday parties from the time they began public school together. She didn't play with all of them equally, but she felt it was important to be inclusive. I think this came from not always being invited to their get-togethers. As a parent, I often heard about birthday parties because other parents looked for carpool arrangements. I was saddened to hear of parties that Jaclyn was not invited to, given by girls I knew she considered to be friends. She certainly had her closest friends that she played with, at our house and their houses too. But I used to wonder, *Don't we, as parents, want our children to learn lessons about inclusion?* I saw the laughter, the camaraderie, and the fun other children had when they came to our house to play with Jaclyn. She would have been overjoyed to receive invitations to their houses as well. Children with illness want to be included too.

I do not mean to infer that Jaclyn or our family lived an isolated existence. We have always had numerous family gatherings and social outings with friends. There were many times that we had to turn down invitations due to illness, but we always knew we had family members and friends who were there for us. Social relationships with friends were a bit more difficult those first few years of Jaclyn's life because kids are sick a lot. If we knew that our nieces or children of family friends were ill, then we often cancelled plans. A cold for another child often became a respiratory infection for Jaclyn, so it wasn't worth the risk. It was during Jaclyn's early school years, when children played on sports teams, that we didn't necessarily feel as if we "fit in." No one particularly excluded us, but our life for many years focused on health, and consequently we were somewhat isolated because of it.

Lessons Jaclyn Taught Me.

Be inclusive. Make lots of friends. Don't keep track of whose turn it is to host the play date. Just play.

Telling Jaclyn About Her Heart

For years, my husband and I agonized over the appropriate time to tell Jaclyn the details about her heart. At what age would she be able to understand? How much should we tell, without scaring her? When she was almost three, before her third surgery, we explained to her that her heart didn't grow the way it was supposed to grow and that a doctor was going to fix it. That seemed to be age-appropriate information.

When she was better able to verbalize, we talked about how some babies are born with parts of their bodies that don't work right. Some of those problems can be fixed, while others cannot. She didn't begin to ask intense questions until age eight, in third grade.

Before age eight, whenever Jaclyn required a cardiac catheterization, or any other procedure, we would tell her two or three days beforehand that she would be going to the hospital. We didn't want to tell her too far in advance because we didn't want her to have nightmares about it. Also, at young ages she did not have a good understanding of time, so it made little sense to tell her much before the actual date.

However, as she approached first and second grade, she asked more questions. She wanted to know how long she would be in the hospital and if she would need to have an IV. We would explain what each procedure would do, in very basic terms. I recall getting myself geared up to tell her of an upcoming cardiac catheterization in which mesh metal stents would be placed into her lung arteries and then ballooned open. It would require one night in the hospital. I was nervous about telling her. Jaclyn asked when it would be, who would be there with her, and then asked if we could play a game. That was it. She got the information she needed from me and then was content to go on about her day.

In third grade, things changed. A school contest had been announced, asking children to reflect and write about "A Different Kind of Hero." Jaclyn had the idea of writing about her surgeon. Her essay was about the surgeon who was a hero because he "saves lives, fixes children's hearts, and checks on them when they are in the hospital." She outlined the paper she would write. I was so proud of her.

Suddenly, Jaclyn wanted to know more about her heart. I realized I needed to explain to her how a "normal" heart develops first, before I could venture into how her heart was different. I put a movie on for my sons, while Jaclyn and I went upstairs to "have a chat" as she called it. In our home office, we have file folders filled with information about Jaclyn's heart—diagrams, research articles, insurance claims, letters from doctors, second opinions, and past hospital and doctor bills. An entire drawer of a file cabinet is reserved solely for this type of information.

I pulled out drawings of hearts. Some were handouts from books and research articles, others were hand-drawn by Jaclyn's surgeon. First I explained basic cardiac anatomy. I walked Jaclyn through the dynamics of a normal heart. I pointed out the aorta, the pulmonary artery, and the four chambers of a heart. I taught her how blood flows from the body to the heart through veins. I explained that the blood circulates through the heart to become oxygenated in the lungs and then travels back to the body via arteries. I remember watching her finger trace the path the blood takes, from blue blood to oxygenated red blood. She understood.

I then described to Jaclyn how her heart was different. I started by pointing to the pulmonary artery and explaining that she simply was born without one. I told her that her first two surgeries (unifocalizations) provided her body with a way to get blood to her lungs, since she wasn't born with the artery necessary to do this. I also showed her pictures of her aorta, located on the opposite side of the heart from where it was supposed to be. I put my finger on the middle of the four chambers of the heart and explained that she had a hole there. We talked about how the blue blood and red blood aren't supposed to mix in the heart, but that hers mixed because there was a hole. I showed her that the tips of my fingers were pinkish. Then we looked at her fingers and noticed that they had a blue tint to them, "because your blood mixes," I explained.

After almost ninety minutes of discussion, I thought we were done for one day. I was psychologically worn out from all her questions—and they were good questions, but I didn't want to go too far. However, Jaclyn wanted to know more. I didn't want her to feel that I wouldn't answer more questions, so I simply told her that I had to tend to the boys and make dinner. I assured her that we would talk more that night, that Daddy could also answer her questions, and that she could ask either of us anything she wanted, anytime.

After dinner that night, Jaclyn and I went back upstairs to the office, took out the pictures again, and resumed our "chat." She wanted to know how the surgeon fixed her heart. I took another deep breath and began to explain the best that I could. I told her that he had joined her tiny arteries together on each side of her lungs into bigger arteries. I explained that he had to re-route the blood around her heart because her aorta was on the wrong side. She wanted to know how.

We talked about roadblocks and how, during construction, vehicles often have to take different routes to get to where they are going. I showed her, on diagrams, how the surgeon had built "new paths" for her blood to flow through. She also wanted to know about the synthetic pieces the surgeon had used to fix her heart over the years. We discussed Gortex, the material that some of her arteries and patches were made of. I recall telling her to think of her pink raincoat; it was made of Gortex. I explained that Gortex was used because it was waterproof, just like her coat, and that it was strong enough to hold the blood without allowing leakage. That explanation would suffice. After another forty minutes of talking, we were both tired.

Each night, Jaclyn was given time to read quietly to herself or to read chapter books with me. That night, after two-plus hours of "chatting" about her heart, she didn't want to read. Instead, she must have pondered what we had discussed. The next night after dinner, Jaclyn took out a piece of paper. On it, she had written fabulous questions that she had thought of the night before. "Why can doctors fix some problems but not others?" "How do doctors know how to fix hearts?" "What other things will have to be fixed in my heart?"

Many days and many chats later, my son, Ryan, wanted to hear what we had been discussing. Jaclyn felt this was a private issue. Ryan wanted to know about it too, but Jaclyn found this unacceptable. Ryan was five years old. I told him that when he was older he could learn about hearts too. I didn't want to discount his interest, but at that time I felt Jaclyn's need for privacy was more important. Ryan was content to know that he would hear about hearts "someday."

Jaclyn wrote the first two paragraphs of that paper on why her surgeon was a hero. Then it occurred to her that if she won, the story would be distributed throughout the school district. "Does this mean everyone in my whole school will know about my heart?" she asked. I told her that her heart was nothing to be ashamed of and that it was not her fault that it hadn't fully developed. I also explained that many of her teachers already knew that her heart was different. I reminded her that when she had been hospitalized in kindergarten (to have her gall bladder removed), her whole class made her a "Get Well Soon" banner. I was hinting that some of her friends already knew a little bit about her heart needing to be fixed and that it was not something she needed to hide or to be embarrassed about.

Jaclyn wanted to think about whether to enter the contest or not. We left it up to her to decide. After a few days of consideration, she decided not to enter the contest. She never finished writing the story about how her surgeon was a hero. She threw the first two paragraphs away. I secretly dug the paper out of the garbage and put it away. I was still very proud of the story she had begun.

Lessons Jaclyn Taught Me.

Even children have a right to medical information, as long as it's age-appropriate. At young ages, discussions about Jaclyn's heart were short, not very detailed, and aimed directly at her questions. We didn't tell her more than she wanted to know. As she aged, her desire for information and her intelligent questions guided our conversations. Alan and I were open to discuss anything, anytime with her, and I know she appreciated our availability and honesty.

Here We Go Again!

For years, Jaclyn and our family didn't think about surgeries or hospitals. We just lived our lives. She had cardiology check-ups every six months. From the time she was six years old, we were "on alert" that another surgery might be imminent because her donated pulmonary valve and artery might be too small for her body, depending on how much she had grown. There was also the possibility that the synthetic pieces would be less functional by that time. But there were no big growth spurts, so surgery wasn't needed yet.

When Jaclyn was 9 ½, she had her standard cardiac check-up. She had been on a growth hormone for six months at that time, and she was indeed growing. In fact, she had grown one and one half inches those first six months on the medication. At this December check-up, the cardiologist discovered that her valve was leaking and needed to be replaced.

The open-heart surgery was not an emergency but did need to be done soon. My first thought was to wait until summer vacation to minimize the amount of fourth grade Jaclyn would miss. The cardiologist said it could not wait that long and that a catheterization would need to be completed first.

The cardiac catheterization took place in January, 2006, to see how bad the leakage was, where it was, and how high the pressures were in Jaclyn's arteries. For years, Jaclyn had had dangerously high pressures. It would have been risky for her to undergo surgery under these conditions. She had been put on a new medication in first grade to try to control these pressures, and fortunately this helped. Her pressures were still high, but not as extreme.

During the cardiac catheterization, the cardiologist determined that Jaclyn's pressures were down even more than he expected. This was good news. However, he also discovered that she had an arrhythmia, an irregular fast heartbeat. This wasn't the first time she had experienced this. The doctor consulted with the surgeon and decided the arrhythmia should be addressed prior to surgery. We were referred to one of only a handful of pediatric electrophysiologists (EP) in Illinois. An EP focuses on heart rhythms and the electrical conductivity of the heart.

Nurses had asked Jaclyn what she felt when the arrhythmia occurred. She said, "It [my heart] feels jumpy." When asked if she ever felt this before, she said she had. We were advised to be sure Jaclyn understood the importance of telling us when she felt the "jumpiness" without making her nervous about it.

We came home and read up on this highly recommended doctor. We also gathered information on ablation, the procedure that would be done to correct the arrhythmia. We wanted to be able to ask intelligent questions upon meeting this doctor.

We took Jaclyn to the appointment and felt comfortable with the doctor immediately. Alan and I had decided that Jaclyn was old enough to hear this consultation. The doctor answered all of our questions, even stopping occasionally to ask Jaclyn if she had questions. He explained how the ablation worked—that he would fish two wires, one through her groin and one through a vessel in her arm, to the heart. He would have to identify the source of the arrhythmia, the location in the conduction system telling the heart to beat an extra time. Once located, he would then ablate, or cauterize, the cells that were sending the irregular message to the heart to beat.

During this meeting he explained a few additional possibilities. The first was that he might not actually be able to do the ablation if he couldn't reach it via catheters. If this turned out to be the case, at least he could provide the surgeon with information about the source of the arrhythmia. The surgeon could then take care of it during the upcoming open-heart surgery. The second possibility he described to us was that, in rare cases ("less than 10%"), heart rates drop after an ablation because the heart no longer beats the extra time. He told us that a pacemaker might be needed to pace Jaclyn's heart and keep it beating at the right speed. At that moment, I looked at the doctor, then at Alan, and said, "Given our experience, even things that might only occur less than 10% of the time often happen to us!" Everybody laughed. The doctor was convinced that Jaclyn would not need a pacemaker, but he was happy to discuss it further with us "just to be prepared."

The nurse got a pacemaker to show us. It was about the size of a half dollar and was approximately one third of an inch thick. Jaclyn held it in her hand. He described how the pacemaker would be implanted in the fatty tissue under the armpit near the chest wall, if needed. Upon looking at Jaclyn, he noted that she had no fatty tissue. He explained that there would be a way to tuck it under muscles in front of the armpit so it would not be visible, all the while leading us to believe she would most likely not need this device.

The ablation took place February 1, 2006. We expected the procedure to last anywhere from two to four hours. The trickiest part would be mapping the location of the arrhythmia and gathering data regarding the electrical circuitry of Jaclyn's heart. This information would be very useful to the surgeon for the upcoming open-heart surgery, so the doctor expected it to take some time.

Less than two hours later, the electrophysiologist and his nurse came to the waiting room to talk to us. When I first saw them, I whispered to Alan, "he wasn't able to do the ablation. If he had, he wouldn't be done so soon." I was disappointed, and my husband also sensed that I might be correct.

The doctor started to tell us that Jaclyn was fine, that she had done well during the procedure, and that the source of the arrhythmia was, in fact, as he had expected it to be. He had gathered the necessary data for the surgeon. Both of us were waiting for him to tell us the ablation wasn't possible. Instead, he kept talking. I remember waiting for him to say he could not actually ablate the proper cells. Suddenly my husband, mother, mother-in-law, and aunt who had been with us in the waiting room were all smiling. "What did he say?" I asked my husband. "It's done!" he replied. "He did it." A feeling of relief came over me. Finally, he told us Jaclyn's heart rate was fine. It was only a bit slow, and it was sustaining itself. Moreover, he expected it to increase as she woke more from the sedation. "No need for a pacemaker," he said.

Jaclyn awakened quickly from the procedure. We were playing games in ICU right away. She would have to spend one night in the hospital for observation. We sent all our relatives home. Both Alan and I were planning to stay at the hospital overnight with Jaclyn, but at dinner time we realized Jaclyn was fine, so I sent my husband home to be with our sons. The plan was for me to stay with her that night and bring her home the next morning.

Jaclyn and I passed the time playing more games, doing Sudoku puzzles, and watching *The King and I*. I remember that we sang "Shall We Dance" out loud, our favorite song from the musical. When the movie ended around 10:00 pm, we decided to call it a night. I was just about to turn off the light in her room, when her heart monitor alarms sounded. A nurse quickly appeared in the doorway. Jaclyn was fine, and I thought it was a false alarm. We turned off the light. Seconds later, it happened again. This time the monitor in Jaclyn's room showed her heart rate to be in the 60s. This was too low. The rate crept back up to its earlier level, in the 90s. Within five minutes, the alarms were beeping incessantly. The monitor read, "Irregular rhythm." Nurses fussed and turned on the lights. Jaclyn was sitting up in bed, wondering what the ruckus was about! She was feeling all right, and I figured that the leads on her chest had simply fallen off, giving faulty readings. I wasn't concerned.

Then our nurse sat down in a chair watching Jaclyn and the monitor. Jaclyn told me she was okay. She looked comfortable and relaxed, so I didn't become concerned. Every few seconds another nurse, who was watching the heart monitor at the nurses' station, ran to our room to ask how Jaclyn was feeling. Finally, Jaclyn said, "It feels like it [my heart] stops and then starts again." *That* did not sound good! Now I was getting nervous. EKGs of her heart rates and rhythms were being faxed to the electrophysiologist at his home. Her heart rate was dipping into the 60s, but always rose back to the 90s on its own. I asked if it was time for me to call my husband, but the nurses assured me Jaclyn was okay and that there was no emergency.

After an hour of this, with a nurse sitting vigil in our room watching my daughter, I snuck into the hall to ask more questions. I hadn't wanted to leave Jaclyn alone, but I really needed to know what was going on. The "Fellow on Call" in the ICU told me that the electrophysiologist wanted to hang an adrenaline drip by Jaclyn's bed "just in case." If needed, adrenaline would raise her heart rate. This sounded easy enough.

Again, I asked if I should summon Alan back to the hospital. I was told there was still no emergency. I asked for the "worst case scenario." Big mistake. The nurse told me that if Jaclyn's heart rate didn't go back up on its own, that they "would have to externally paddle her." I had heard enough. I called Alan in a panic and told him what had transpired in the last hour and a half. He assured me that if the EP wasn't concerned, we shouldn't be either. Alan asked me to call him back when I knew more. I was a wreck and couldn't believe I was in the hospital alone with Jaclyn during all of this. But again, Jaclyn's demeanor was calm and somewhat relaxing to me.

Shortly after that, the adrenaline drip was started. Within fifteen minutes, Jaclyn's heart rate was up, but now it was almost 120 beats per minute, which was too high. The doctor on call was in constant contact with the electrophysiologist, monitoring all that was happening. They adjusted the dosage of adrenaline, and slowly Jaclyn's heart rate tapered off to about 100 beats per minute, which is where they wanted it to be.

Just before midnight, the electrophysiologist called me on the phone in Jaclyn's room and told me that we couldn't go home without a pacemaker. I asked if it needed to be done in the middle of the night. He informed me that many logistical issues would be worked out and that decisions would be made in the morning. He reminded me that I was the one who guessed that a pacemaker would be needed! It wasn't funny this time.

The logistical issues were complex. First our surgeon didn't know what was happening. There was the possibility that he would want to move up the date of Jaclyn's open-heart surgery. He could then replace the leaking valve and artery and also put in a pacemaker at the same time. But nobody knew if he would want to do all of this in one surgery or two. If he decided the pacemaker surgery should be separate, there was the question of whether that would delay the open-heart surgery, which had already been put off because of the ablation. *How long could the open-heart surgery wait before that too became an emergency?* we wondered. On the contrary, if he wanted to put in a pacemaker and also perform the open-heart surgery the next day, *we* were not ready. We had not yet made arrangements for our boys, and Alan hadn't made arrangements for time off from work. We had anticipated the open-heart surgery necessitating approximately three weeks in the hospital and then additional recovery time at home. We simply were not ready, although it was not even our decision to make.

Another issue was *who* would put in the pacemaker? The electrophysiologist could perform this surgery, but we had come to a closer hospital to have the ablation done. If cardiac complications arose, we were far from our surgeon. We were presented the option of having Jaclyn transported by ambulance to our regular hospital to have the pacemaker put in.

It was midnight when I called Alan and told him to pack our suitcase with a few days worth of clothes. I explained that Jaclyn was fine, but that she could not come home without a pacemaker, as her heart rate was too slow. I told him additional decisions would be made in the morning, when the EP consulted with the cardiac surgeon. Fortunately, when he had gone home that evening, my mom had had the foresight to sleep at our house, "just in case." Alan woke her up to tell her he was returning to the hospital, and she stayed with Ryan and Joshua.

The next morning, we learned that the surgeon did *not* want to do the open-heart surgery yet. He wanted the pacemaker put in and for Jaclyn to heal before the open-heart surgery was scheduled. He was confident we could stay at the hospital we were at and have the electrophysiologist put in the pacemaker. The whole idea of transporting by ambulance to another hospital made me nervous anyway. So we stayed and had the EP insert the pacemaker.

The electrophysiologist was en route to another hospital when he got the call to return to put in Jaclyn's pacemaker. His nurse and his choice of anesthesiologist were also called to the hospital. An operating room would have to be made available, and we were told the pacemaker would probably not be put in until late in the afternoon or in the evening. Meanwhile, Jaclyn took all of this with a grain of salt and was mostly concerned about the few added days of school she would miss. Her attitude was great once again. Meanwhile, I was a nervous wreck.

She remained on the adrenaline drip and was doing fine.

We would not be going home that morning after all. She would be having an unplanned surgery to place a pacemaker, and hopefully we could be discharged the next day. She was not allowed to eat or drink anything because nobody knew what time her surgery would be. This was difficult, but there was nothing that could be done about it. I couldn't believe that my premonition about the pacemaker was coming true.

At 11:00 am, the electrophysiologist came to say the procedure would begin just after noon. Normally, a pacemaker is placed in the armpit or the chest cavity on the left side of the body because it is closer to the heart. But because Jaclyn is left-handed, the doctor put the pacemaker in her right chest instead. Placing the actual devise was the easy part. Fishing the pacing lead to the heart and finding a spot on the heart with good electrical conductivity was more of a challenge.

When Jaclyn woke up, she had a two-inch incision in front of her right armpit. Otherwise, she felt fine. Recovery was more than we had planned for; after all, she originally came in only to have an ablation. We were able to go home the next day. But to ensure that the pacing lead could fully implant itself into the heart's wall, Jaclyn was not to lift her right arm above her shoulder, or to carry any weight in that arm, for six weeks. She wore a sling to remind herself and others to be careful of her right arm. She could not participate in gym class or have recess for six weeks either. All in all, she had the ablation on a Wednesday, the pacemaker was put in on Thursday, and she returned to school Monday. What a trooper!

With the pacemaker came the addition of two more medications to our regime. Jaclyn now required Coumadin, a blood thinner, as well as baby aspirin. She was up to twelve doses of medication each day. With Coumadin came the need to have a blood test every four to six weeks to ascertain whether she had the appropriate amount of the blood thinner in her body. Jaclyn despised blood tests. And there were certain symptoms that we now had to watch for in her. As long as she had a pacemaker, we had to be wary of fevers above 102 degrees because that could indicate a reaction to the foreign device in her body. In addition, I was given a card to carry in my wallet identifying my daughter as a pacemaker wearer, since she would no longer be able to walk through security systems without setting off alarms. We were also warned about the potential for bleeding with Jaclyn now on these two blood thinning medications. We were told that normal cuts and scrapes would probably bleed more than normal and that bruising would likely be more severe. Jaclyn had occasional nose bleeds from the oxygen she slept with at night. Luckily, we didn't notice much of a difference. But administering her growth hormone injections would now cause bruises up and down her thighs because of these two new medications. Again, she took this all in stride.

The surgeon wanted to wait at least six weeks for Jaclyn to heal before the open-heart surgery. We scheduled it right before spring vacation so she would miss a bit less school. We now had a date, and preparations began in earnest. Jaclyn wore a Snoopy and Peanuts sling on her right arm, had a new scar needing to heal, couldn't do some things, but otherwise she didn't let any of this slow her down. She continued her school work, played with friends after school, and bombarded us with requests to play games with her at home.

This Surgery Is Completely Different

For six weeks Jaclyn rode the elevator at school and had a buddy carry her backpack for her. She had difficulty climbing stairs because of the catheter that had been in her leg, she couldn't participate in recess or physical education class, and she couldn't lift her right arm or carry anything. At first Jaclyn came home from school at lunch and recess time. We watched game shows on television and played board games before she'd return to school for the afternoon. Then her Girl Scout troop set up a schedule so that two friends would stay indoors with her during recess each day. The school and her friends were going out of their way to help. It was very touching.

I met with Jaclyn's teachers to talk about the upcoming surgery and the anticipated missed school. Academically, Jaclyn was in great shape. However, it had been a long time since she had endured open-heart surgery. I didn't know what to expect this time. Her last open-heart surgery was at age three, and she was in the hospital for over three weeks. It took months for her to regain her strength and endurance once she came home from the hospital. I was worried that this time she could potentially miss six to eight weeks of school, depending upon how things went.

This surgery would be very different though for many reasons. First, Jaclyn was older and, consequently, she better understood what was happening this time. Second, she was bigger, but her heart had been enlarged over the years from high pressures and having to work extra hard. A third difference was that we now had two other children. Ryan and Joshua hadn't been born when Jaclyn had her first four heart surgeries. Logistically, having the boys presented huge challenges. Finally, Jaclyn would potentially be missing a good amount of fourth grade. She had many friends and didn't want to continuously talk about the surgery with them, although she wanted them to know why she wasn't at recess to play Four-Square, why she wasn't sitting with her regular group in the school cafeteria for lunch, and why her desk was empty.

I wanted the teachers to send home school assignments that Jaclyn would be missing in March and April. But there wasn't much work we could do in advance. I met with the school principal to discuss the missed school. I was told that our school district would provide a tutor for Jaclyn when she was feeling up to it. I kept that notion in the back of my mind, though I felt that I could just as easily do the work with Jaclyn myself after she recuperated, since she was so motivated and in good academic standing anyway.

I began to make a "Master Calendar" as I lined up various friends and neighbors to help take care of Ryan and Joshua. We explained to the boys that Jaclyn would be in the hospital for surgery and that we would not be coming home for the first few days. They knew they would be cared for by various people and that they would be spending many days going to different friends' houses. I encouraged them to tell me whose houses they wanted to go to, and I tried to call those friends for favors. Ryan was in first grade, so he was in school every day from 9:00 am to 3:35 pm. Joshua only attended preschool two mornings per week, from 9:00–11:30 am. He was home with me the rest of the time. So I had a multitude of babysitting arrangements to coordinate.

I had Ryan being taken to school and picked up from school by different people each day. Joshua needed to be driven to and from preschool. On the days he didn't have school, I arranged for him to play at a friend's house in the morning and then I had that friend drive him to the next house for the afternoon. That person would, in turn, bring Joshua home when a relative could be at my house to stay with both boys. I had different people feeding the boys their dinner and putting them to bed. And although I tried, for consistency, to have the same people sleep at my house with them each night, it didn't always work out that way. On the weekends, I coordinated play dates where both boys could go to the same house together. My Master Calendar was overwhelming. Two weeks before surgery, I was having anxiety about how chaotic life would be for them. I felt terrible that I wouldn't see them for a few days and that I couldn't even tell them what day we would be home. I was crying every time friends asked how I was holding up.

Meanwhile, Jaclyn asked lots of questions about the surgery. "How long will I be asleep?" "Will you be there when I wake up?" "How long will I be on the ventilator?" "Can I talk to you while on the vent?" "How many IVs will I need, and can they be put in *after* I'm asleep?" "When can I go back to school?" "Will I miss the school talent show later in the school year?" "How many Girl Scout meetings will I miss?" "When can I play the piano again?"

Although we answered all her questions, we knew she still didn't really understand the complexity and seriousness of this surgery. We didn't want to frighten her. However, we did explain that she would be unable to speak when on the ventilator, that she would sleep for many days as her body healed, and that she would have many IVs and monitors in both arms and also in her groin. We told her she would be in the hospital for a few weeks, not days, like she was used to for the smaller procedures she could remember. We reminded her that she might be sore and that she might need assistance doing the things she used to do by herself, until she fully recovered.

Preparations also included soliciting blood donors for the surgery. We were asked to have four units of blood donated. We asked neighbors, friends, and Alan's work colleagues to donate blood. I had learned from past experience that donors are sometimes turned away on the day of donation for various reasons—they might be sick, they might have traveled to one of the many countries that make one's blood questionable according to the blood bank, or they might be anemic. So I assembled six donors instead of the requested four.

I was to be one of the directed donors, as my blood type matches Jaclyn's. I had donated blood for each of her past surgeries. But this time, I broke down crying in the clinic on the day I was to give my blood. The nurses saw how emotional I was and advised against me donating.

We knew that if Jaclyn even had a drippy nose, the surgery

would be cancelled and rescheduled at a later time. In addition to his full-time job, Alan was now attending graduate school on alternate weekends to earn his MBA. We had purposely picked the surgery date of March 13th because it was one week before Jaclyn's spring vacation, which meant she would miss one less week of school. Alan also had a weekend without graduate school during that time of year. However, if surgery needed to be rescheduled due to illness, we would lose the luxury of that extra week off. In the back of our minds, we also thought that by having the surgery in mid-March we were assuring that Jaclyn would be home from the hospital in time for her tenth birthday on May 6th. We had a lot riding on that date and had made all the necessary preparations.

Two weeks before surgery, lots of kids in school were sick. After all, it was winter in Chicago. Jaclyn's teachers were very accommodating and switched her classroom seat on a daily basis so she would not be sitting next to someone who was sniffling or coughing or next to someone who had just returned to school after illness. At home, I became fanatical about germs. As soon as anyone came into my house, they washed their hands. When the kids came home from school at the end of the day, I made them change their clothes. I wiped doorknobs and telephones. I'm sure I was a pain to live with during that time. I had arrangements lined up for the boys, and I didn't want to have to redo my Master Calendar if a new surgery date was needed. I had blood donors scheduled to donate. If they gave their blood, and then Jaclyn got sick, the blood would no longer be fresh, and I'd have to start soliciting donors again. As far as I was concerned, March 13th had to materialize.

The week before surgery, I decided to keep Jaclyn home from school. Even her teachers concurred that the classroom was a cesspool of germs. So Jaclyn and I hung out at home together. As usual we played a lot of games. We made crafts. We watched game shows on television, and she began to do all the homework she would be missing over the next many weeks of missed school.

In one week's time, Jaclyn and I were able to plow through much of her homework. She liked school so it wasn't a problem to work on assignments for hours at a time. She tackled math first because it was her favorite subject. She even got ahead. We did science experiments at home on electricity, as the school sent home the needed equipment and supplies. We completed an entire book on Map Essentials, twenty assignments in all, in less than a week. She worked on spelling and grammar homework. She was in good shape, which made me feel more relaxed about the amount of school she would be missing. She had gotten far ahead in one week, so I knew it would be possible to make up whatever else she would miss.

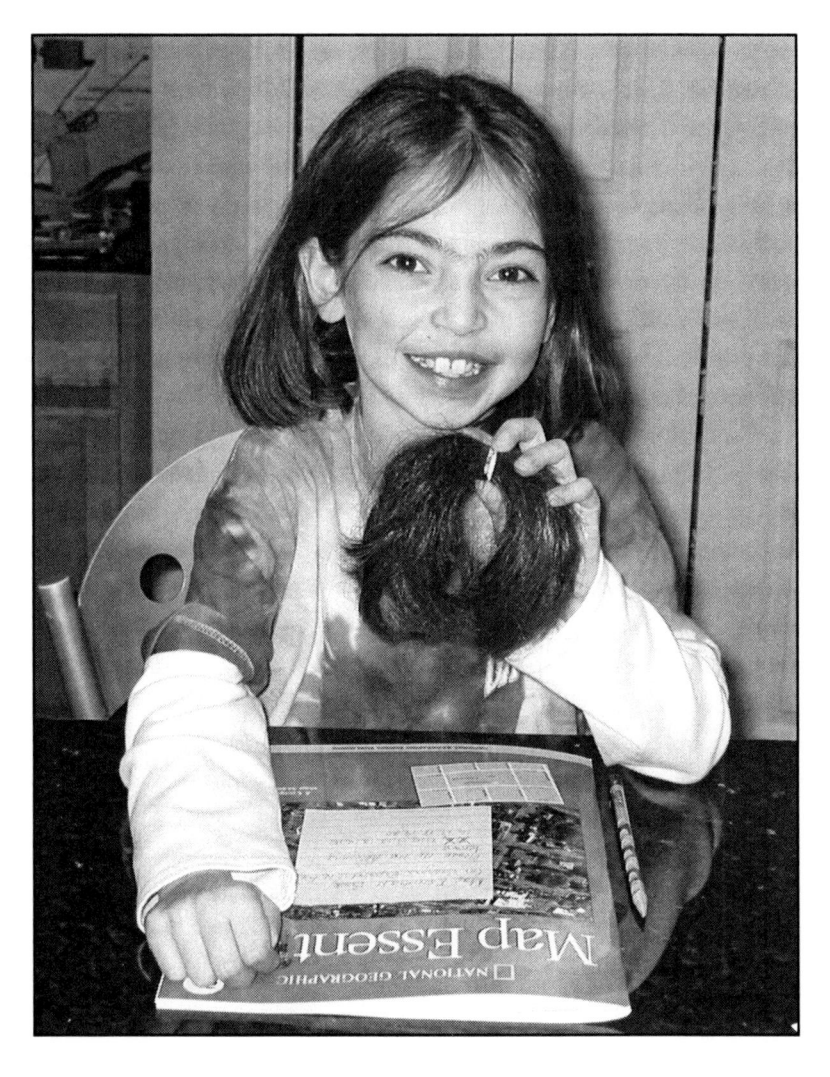

After we cut Jaclyn's hair, in preparation for upcoming surgery, she shows off the ponytail she donated to Locks of Love, (March, 2006).

One day it occurred to me that Jaclyn's long hair should be cut prior to surgery. I remembered how difficult it had been to wash and bathe her in a hospital bed when she was younger. Her incisions could not get wet, and long hair made it more difficult. She was quarantined at home, so instead of taking her to a salon I cut her hair myself. I had never done that before. I did my best to cut about seven inches off the bottom of her hair, making it shoulder-length. As we were gathering up the loose hair, Jaclyn told me she had an idea. She had read in *Time Magazine for Kids* that children with cancer often wear wigs after their hair falls out from chemotherapy. She knew that people could donate their hair to be made into wigs for these children. She asked if she could donate her hair for that cause. We immediately searched the internet and found "Locks of Love," an organization that accepts donated hair to be used in wigs. Luckily, we had just enough hair in her collected ponytail to meet their requirements. She sent in a full ponytail of her hair with a note, and she was proud to receive a certificate of thanks months later.

Meanwhile, I had been so busy with my juggling act of things to do before the surgery that I realized I hadn't paid attention to my own fears about what Jaclyn would be going through. I had too many balls in the air—arrangements for the boys, Jaclyn's homework, trying to fit special activities in for Ryan and Joshua, blood donors, relatives coming into town to help us, and making sure to try to spend quality time with each child. My husband was busy completing projects for work in anticipation of a three-week leave of absence. Plus, he was studying for finals for his MBA. Life was chaotic. But we tried our best to make it as "normal" for the kids as we could, even though talk of "hospitals" and "surgery" popped up a lot.

Last-Minute Hassles

The day before surgery, nerves were flaring throughout our house. Jaclyn had been in quarantine, so she had not seen anyone for a week. However, against my better judgment, many people came to our house the day before surgery to give Jaclyn "a quick kiss." My in-laws came into town to help take care of the boys. My mom and cousin came to sleep over, since they would be needed the next morning to get the boys to school. My aunt poked her head in the door to kiss Jaclyn and to tell her to "be tough." There was a lot of activity that day, despite our desire to make it as mellow as we could.

Jaclyn had to be admitted to the hospital on Sunday night for a Monday morning surgery. Alan, Jaclyn and I packed our bags, hugged and kissed the boys and grandparents goodbye, and headed to the hospital. We were admitted to a regular pediatric room. Jaclyn's medical history was taken, and she volunteered to tell the nurse the names and dosages of all her medications. She even spelled them correctly when the nurse could not. The nurse was impressed.

Throughout the admission, Jaclyn sat in her hospital bed filling out NCAA brackets for the upcoming college tournament. It was March, and the top sixty-four teams were being announced as we sat in her room. As a sports fanatic, she wanted to know how the Fighting Illini from the University of Illinois were ranked and what team they would be playing in Round One. The nurse seemed amused.

There had been discussion back and forth for days before

the surgery about whether Jaclyn should continue taking the growth hormones during the surgical recovery. The endocrinologist who prescribed them advised stopping the medicine because a potential side effect was fluid retention. This tended to be a problem Jaclyn encountered after past surgeries.

However, the orders written on the medical chart were to give the growth hormone. We explained why the endocrinologist counseled us against this, and the nurse took the information to the doctor on call. This doctor, who didn't know us or our daughter and didn't even come in to meet us, told the nurse to skip the growth hormone dosage for Sunday night, but that it could resume Monday after surgery. This was ludicrous because, as we explained, the drug could cause fluid retention. He brushed our comments aside and simply wrote the order to give the growth hormone on Monday. Alan and I planned to discuss it with the surgeon the next day.

Meanwhile, Jaclyn had been taking Coumadin, a blood thinning medication, since receiving the pacemaker a month earlier. However, blood thinners must be stopped prior to surgery due to the risk of bleeding. Her last dose was given Saturday night, two days before surgery. For safety, the surgeon still wanted her to receive a blood thinner, but one that was shorter-acting. This was the reason Jaclyn had to be admitted to the hospital on Sunday night. She was to be started on an IV heparin drip at 5:00 pm. The IV was to be stopped in the middle of the night so it would be out of her system by the time surgery was to begin on Monday at 7:30 am.

Alan and I slept in the room with Jaclyn. At midnight we were awakened by the nurse. She informed us that she had misread the admission orders regarding the heparin. She was supposed to have given Jaclyn a large dose of the blood thinner upon starting the IV drip at 5:00 pm on Sunday, and then taper the dosage gradually. It was to be turned off completely at 3:00 am. However, the nurse had not given the large dose, and instead Jaclyn had only been receiving the minimal amount over seven hours. The nurse apologized for the error and said a blood test would be needed to identify how much heparin was actually in Jaclyn's body. Obviously, the appropriate amount wouldn't be in her system, and so the blood test seemed like a waste of time. Sure enough, Jaclyn had only half the amount in her body that she was supposed to have.

The nurse proceeded to rectify the problem by giving the large dosage of the blood thinner at 1:30 am. The drip was to be turned off completely in ninety minutes. I realized there was nothing that could be done about the fact that Jaclyn had not received the right amount of the medication. However, it made no sense to increase her dose so close to the time the IV was to be stopped. After all, the blood thinner was supposed to be out of her system only six hours later! I had specifically been told at Jaclyn's pre-operative visit two days earlier, by both a nurse and a doctor, to be sure the IV drip was turned off at 3:00 am! The seriousness of this request was well understood on my part. So I refused to allow the large dose to be given.

I asked to speak to a doctor. It was the middle of the night Monday morning. The doctor on call at 1:30 am was the same man who had previously brushed us off regarding growth hormones and their potential for causing fluid retention. He was the one who told the nurse to rectify her error by giving the large dose of heparin. I wanted our surgeon to make the decision, not this doctor who had already lost my trust earlier in the evening.

The surgeon's assistant was called, and the message was relayed to us. It was now 2:00 am. This surgical assistant explained that if excessive blood thinner was found to be in Jaclyn's system at 7:30 am, at the time surgery was to begin, another drug could be administered to reverse the effect. Why hadn't someone told us this at midnight? If the doctor on call had explained this to us, there would have been less concern about giving Jaclyn the large dose. Instead, we were not given this information, and needless to say, nobody slept that night.

For the record, the surgeon adamantly refused to resume Jaclyn's growth hormone injections after surgery and during recovery. I had been right to raise the issue with the doctor on call. That validation was very comforting.

Lessons Jaclyn Taught Me.

Neither Alan nor I have medical training. However, we have been told over the years that we have come to know and understand a lot about our daughter's medical condition. As parents of a chronically ill child, it seemed crucial for us to educate ourselves, as best we could, about

Jaclyn's heart anatomy. While I never set out to purposely question a doctor's authority, there were definitely times when I insisted on learning more and asking further questions to better understand. Jaclyn's cardiologist learned to expect a slew of questions from me because he knew my style was to gather information and educate myself.

With a medically fragile child, I believe it is IMPERATIVE for parents to feel comfortable to ask questions of their doctors. And in this case, I felt validated to know that I had been correct about the growth hormone and the urgency of the blood thinning medication being out of Jaclyn's body prior to the start of surgery. I couldn't be shy around doctors while my child's well-being was at stake. I wasn't questioning the judgment of the on call doctor; I was simply reiterating what I had been told by our surgeon at a preoperative visit days earlier. I've learned that it's important for me to be confident that I understand what is happening. If I do not understand, I ask. And in this case, I'm so glad I did. Health care professionals can do better in terms of making parents feel comfortable asking questions and raising issues.

The reason for my steadfastness in this area was that I knew Jaclyn would someday be responsible for her own doctors' appointments. I surmised that she would learn, in part from Alan and me, how to interact with the people who took care of her. I wanted her to feel empowered to ask questions, get clarification, and handle differing opinions from health professionals. I spoke up on her behalf because I wanted her to be able to do the same for herself in the future.

Fifth Open-Heart Surgery (and an Emergency Sixth!)

It was hard to sleep the night before surgery, despite knowing that it would be beneficial to get some rest. But on those nights I found myself talking to G-d a lot, peeking at Jaclyn over and over, and trying not to think too much!

On Monday morning, we walked Jaclyn to the surgical recovery room where we would say our goodbyes. It was always hard not to get emotional at these times, as I didn't want to make Jaclyn more afraid than she already was. This was actually the first surgery that she expressed being scared. She was now old enough to understand what was happening, which made it so much harder on us. She was given oral medicine to make her groggy, but she fought it. When the nurses and anesthesiologist were ready to wheel her bed into the operating room, there were tears in her eyes. It was one of many awful moments we, as parents, have had to endure. She reminded us one more time to "be there" when she awoke.

We walked alongside her bed as far as we were allowed to go. We kissed her again, I stroked her head and wiped her tears. I whispered to "be tough" and reminded her that she'd "be okay." Then the nurses pushed her through doors marked "Authorized Personnel Only." My husband and I stood hugging for many minutes, staring at the closed door.

The surgeon had told us that this surgery would be "very long." When asked to clarify what that meant, we were told "it could take all day." Jaclyn still had high pressures in her lungs because her heart was working hard to pump through vessels that were too small. The goals of the surgery were fourfold. First, replace the leaking pulmonary valve. Second, exchange the donated artery that had been placed into her heart when she was three years old with a new synthetic one. Third, enlarge the arteries going to her lungs via a patch. And fourth, attach a second pacemaker lead to her heart for use "down the road, if ever needed."

The physician's assistant updated us throughout the surgery, as she did during all previous surgeries. She came to the family waiting room after about an hour to tell us Jaclyn was prepped and that they were about to begin. Every sixty to ninety minutes she would provide more information about what had already been accomplished and what was to come next. We were always given a time frame for when her next update would be. She never let us down.

After eleven grueling hours of sitting in that family waiting room, watching other family members of patients come and go, Jaclyn's surgery was over, and she was doing well. We had kissed her goodbye just before 8:00 am that morning. The first time we got to see her in her PSHU room was 7:45 pm. As usual, the first time I entered her room I had to catch my breath. The machines, the IVs, the medications and the ventilator were, again, overwhelming to me. I started to cry. I cried because I hated to see my daughter that way. At some point I realized that the surgery was over, and I cried even harder out of relief.

Having not slept the night before and having experienced the stress of eleven hours of waiting, we were exhausted. We were relieved too but definitely over-tired. We knew that the first night after surgery was our best opportunity to actually sleep, as Jaclyn would be heavily sedated and "paralyzed."

Over the years I have heard the surgeon and nurses use the word "paralyzed" to describe a child, post-surgery. It meant that the patient would be given medication disabling him/her from movement. Right after surgery, the body requires rest. This medication was administered to allow healing to begin. I have always felt a jolt of anxiety upon hearing that word although I understood its purpose. Even though she couldn't hear us, we spent a few hours with Jaclyn, talking to her, reminding her that it was over, and whispering to her to get a good night's sleep. After staying with her until we could barely keep our eyes open, we went to bed. During this surgery in 2006, the Guest House no longer existed, as the hospital was fundraising to build a Ronald McDonald House for families to use during their child's hospitalization. So this first night, we did something we had never done during past surgeries—we did not both stay with Jaclyn in her hospital room. My mom and I slept at a hotel down the street from the hospital, and Alan slept in the hospital waiting room.

We had been prepared for Day Two to be a "sleeping and healing day," and that's what we had told Jaclyn. But she had other plans. On the day after surgery, she had begun to awaken from the sedation, and though groggy, she was desperate to communicate with us. Before the surgery, we had reminded her that she would be on a ventilator when she woke up and that she would be unable to talk. She asked if she could write notes to us. Because we thought she'd be too sleepy, we told her that wouldn't work. The day after surgery, she was in her PSHU bed half-asleep, her body motionless except for a waving hand. She was waving her arm in the air, but her hand was trying to grasp something. I remembered the earlier request about writing and realized she was asking for paper and a pencil.

A nurse brought the desired supplies, but by then Jaclyn was sleeping again. Next time she woke, she motioned again. This time we were ready. Jaclyn is left-handed. But her left hand was inaccessible, attached to a board with multiple IVs taped to it. Also, she was lying on her left side. Her right arm was all that was free. This was the arm that waved; the only part of her body, in fact, that moved. With eyes closed, she tried to write a message to us on paper. She kept writing in the same place on the paper, new letters covering old ones. And using her right hand, despite being left-handed, made it completely illegible.

Next, I had the idea for Jaclyn to form letters with her finger instead of with a pencil. We still could not make heads or tails out of what she was trying to tell us. We assumed it had to do with the ventilator and when it would be coming out, but we had already answered all those questions. She obviously had something else to say. Frustrated, she closed her eyes and drifted back to sleep.

Hours later she woke and tried again. This time I focused solely on the movement her finger was making on the paper to try and ascertain what letter she was trying to form. I paid no attention to the end result of her writing, but rather on how her finger was moving. After painstaking efforts to understand, I realized she was saying, "When drink?" The answer was that she couldn't have a drink for hours, maybe days, depending how long she was on the ventilator. Another request: "bathroom." She didn't realize she had been catheterized or what that meant. We explained, but she kept spelling the word "bathroom." She didn't like the idea of urinating in the bed, or that in fact, she had been using the catheter for hours already, unbeknownst to her.

On Tuesday night, she was still writing messages to us, more clearly now with a pencil, though still using her right hand. "Very hot." "Time?" "When tube out?" We told her that it was still Tuesday and that it was a "resting day." She hated hearing that the ventilator would be in until the next day, at the earliest. Then she'd fall back asleep, and when she woke again, her first question would be "Time?" She had no concept of whether a few minutes, hours, or a whole day had passed. Later she wrote "Pick 4." Neither Alan nor I could figure out what that meant. Then she made her hand dance. I figured out that she wanted to hear a CD, *Kids' Picks: Mix 4*. She dozed in and out of wakefulness that whole day and night. A whole day and night that we had expected her to be fast asleep.

By Wednesday morning, she was writing longer sentences, more often. Because she was receiving less sedation, her writing was more legible. "How many hours 'til I can drink?" "How long tube in?" "How can I go to the bathroom?" "Dad." "Mom." "Hungry."

While we thought it was wonderful that she was so alert and able to communicate with us, the nurses were shocked. They had never witnessed any child communicating this way. No one could believe that Jaclyn was awake, but not violently fighting the ventilator. In their experience, those hours of wakefulness for a child slowly being weaned from a ventilator were awful. When Jaclyn was a baby and toddler, watching her during those hours *was* horrible. But we had prepared her for the ventilator, and she understood this time that fighting it wouldn't make it go away any faster. Instead, she accepted that it was just part of the recovery and dealt with it the best she could. Different nurses kept poking their heads into our PSHU room to watch Jaclyn, half awake, half asleep, writing voraciously on a clipboard. "What an amazing child!" was uttered over and over again by nurses, residents, respiratory therapists, and anyone who came into her room that day.

Finally, the ventilator was removed late in the day on Wednesday. Less than forty-eight hours since the end of surgery seemed like a blessing to us. Jaclyn was much more comfortable. Now her obsession for a drink began. She had been receiving "maintenance fluids" via IV but hadn't had any food or drink since 10:00 pm Sunday night. When the surgeon came through the PSHU for rounds, Jaclyn asked him when she could have a drink. Her voice was soft, weak and raspy from the ventilator. He gave in and agreed to a few sips of apple juice. The smile on her face lit up the room!

Jaclyn was progressing nicely from the surgery. We were ecstatic. We had hoped for a speedy recovery but knew from past experience that each day often brought new challenges or bumps in the road. On Friday, Jaclyn was doing so well that I went home to see Ryan and Joshua. Neither Alan nor I had been home for five days. I went home and played with Joshua all morning. Then I surprised Ryan by picking him up at school. I made the boys' favorite dinner. Then we got into our pajamas and watched a movie on the floor of the family room. I slept with them that night. They had been concerned about their sister too but handled it well at home with various family members.

The next morning, I headed back to the hospital. Alan was going to come home for his turn to see the boys. Months earlier I had been alone with Jaclyn the night her heart rate had dropped, and the decision was made for her to have a pacemaker. I was actually frightened to be alone with her again, though I hated to admit it. My mom, sensing my insecurity, volunteered to sleep with me at the hospital that night so my husband could go home.

Saturday afternoon, after he left, was a regular day of recovery. Jaclyn was reclining in bed and able to play, make bookmarks out of popsicle sticks, felt and beads, read books, and watch movies. She had been given the okay to eat solid foods. Her first desire was Domino's pizza. I ran out to get her one. It was burnt—a bad omen.

After coming off a ventilator, it usually took Jaclyn awhile, often days, to clear her lungs. She had been encouraged to sit up and cough hard to loosen phlegm in her lungs and chest. But coughing hurt after open-heart surgery. Getting to a sitting position wasn't comfortable, though once she was sitting up, she was fine. Each time she would need to cough, we would have to get her to a sitting position by putting our hands behind her back and slowly pushing her forward. Then to cough, she would hug a soft pillow to her chest. It was painful. We had been doing this for three days.

Saturday night Jaclyn sat up to cough while my mom and I sat beside her. It was just another one of the ordinary coughs she had been making all week. But this time, when she sat up to cough, un-ordinary things were happening! First, I noticed that the top steri-strip, the piece of tape covering her chest incision, was a bit damp. I called a nurse who said that it was common for a bit of oozing to occur through the steri-strips as the incision healed. She was not concerned.

Then Jaclyn coughed with a pillow to her chest. When she put the pillow down, I noticed a drop of blood on it from where it had laid against her chest. This was not right. I saw a droplet of blood on Jaclyn's top steri-strip, at the tip of the incision. I called the nurse again. When we turned on the lights, I was horrified at what I saw!

It looked as if my daughter had swallowed an orange! Her neck was enlarged with a big bulge in it! I yelled for a nurse. She, in turn, called immediately for a doctor. Then things got scary. The more Jaclyn coughed, the more blood started to ooze from her chest incision. And nobody could explain what was happening with her neck. It was now 10:30 pm on a Saturday night. The "Fellow on Call" ordered an ultrasound of Jaclyn's neck. She wanted to be sure Jaclyn's airway was secure. The ultrasound showed no obstruction. Then a chest x-ray was ordered to be sure fluid was not building up around Jaclyn's heart. That x-ray was clear too.

Different nurses and the Fellow kept telling my mother and I that they had never seen anything like this before. It never occurred to anyone that perhaps Jaclyn was bleeding, as all her monitors (heart rate, blood pressure, oxygen saturations) were normal. They surmised that if she was in distress, the monitors would give such an indication. And these machines weren't alarming.

I wanted answers, and nobody could provide them. By 11:00 pm, the entire bandage on Jaclyn's chest was soaked with blood. Even though she was tired, she could not lie back because the swelling in her neck pushed on her airway and was very uncomfortable. She was deliriously exhausted. Meanwhile, the Fellow kept assuring me that she was in contact with the surgeon. He, too, was concerned about the airway but was being told by the Fellow that Jaclyn's breathing wasn't compromised.

At midnight I called Alan. He had gone home for the first time in six days to be with our sons. I woke him and told him he needed to make the hour drive back to the hospital as quickly as possible. At that point there was not a lot of information to share. I told him Jaclyn was bleeding through her incision, that there was a lump in her neck, and that she was exhausted, but couldn't sleep. I tried to hide from him the terror I was feeling.

Alan arrived at the hospital at 1:00 am. The surgeon had been called again, and Jaclyn's neck had been viewed a second time via ultrasound. Still, no answers. The staff, as well as my mother and I, were racking our brains to come up with explanations. We wondered, *Could she be having an allergic reaction to a medication?* Nurses scanned the medical chart and found that no new medications had been started in the last day or so. An allergy to a medication was ruled out. We painstakingly recalled every item of food that Jaclyn had consumed in the last days. Not only had she not eaten anything new, but she had mostly been eating only foods we had brought from home, except for a few bites of the burnt pizza. A food allergy didn't seem to explain this either.

The nurses, residents, and Fellow on Call that were with us were confounded. As a parent of a hospitalized child, it was not comforting to be told that they had no explanation for the swollen neck or the bleeding. I kept asking them to call the surgeon again. The Fellow assured me she was in contact with him and had no new information to present him. I didn't care! I wanted him to know what was happening, and I didn't think it should wait!

To calm me, nurses asked me to leave Jaclyn's bedside. In soothing voices, they reminded me that the more uptight I became, the more nervous Jaclyn would also become. While I understood this, there was no way I could *not* be upset. To me, it looked like very little was actually being done, short of a few ultrasounds, changing her soaked chest bandages, and watching her monitors. I believed that more intense action was called for, and I wasn't satisfied with anything less.

Somewhere in the back of my mind, the fact that Jaclyn was delirious was bothering me too. I knew she was completely exhausted. It had been twenty-two hours since she had slept last. But I was secretly worried that whatever had caused her neck to enlarge might also have affected her brain. I told nobody about these fears. Instead, I tried to ask Jaclyn questions to see if she was really all right. My husband thought I was insane to be asking Jaclyn the name of the Judy Blume book we were currently reading. But I wanted to assess her, and the only way I knew how to do that was to ask her questions. She couldn't answer me. I was petrified, but I convinced myself that she couldn't possibly have brain damage. I talked myself into believing that she was just too tired to answer, or that it was too hard to talk because of her enlarged throat. A part of me was still worried, but I kept it to myself.

Meanwhile, Jaclyn was pale as a ghost! I had never before been more scared. Alan sat in Jaclyn's hospital bed with her. She was sitting between his legs so she could lean against his chest. He was holding her head between his hands, and she was trying to sleep sitting up. Alan sat holding her head for five hours. Jaclyn was exhausted. She couldn't lie down because whatever was in her neck pushed on her throat and her airway. She was pale, and she was now talking in a raspy voice. And blood was *oozing* out of her chest incision!

After hours of watching her, hours of being on edge, the surgeon was summoned to the hospital. It was 5:00 am on Sunday morning. When he arrived, he walked into Jaclyn's PSHU room, and the look on his face was unlike any I had ever seen on him in all the years we had known him! He told us to leave the room immediately. We kissed Jaclyn and went to the waiting room. A few minutes later he came out to tell us he had put Jaclyn back on the ventilator to secure her airway. When we went back to her room, she was sedated and on the ventilator.

My first thought was that Jaclyn would be angry about having been put on the ventilator without being told. We had no idea this was going to happen and hadn't prepared her. I was terribly upset, though I knew it wasn't anyone's fault.

The surgeon was worried that perhaps fluid was gathering around Jaclyn's heart. If this was the case, it would mean her heart wasn't recovering from the surgery and that would be disastrous. He needed our consent to insert a tube into her chest for possible drainage. This had happened to Jaclyn after surgery when she was a toddler. We consented, kissed her again, and left the room. This time, when he came out his face told us there was something else wrong. He expected fluid to come out of the tube he had inserted. Instead, blood came out. And not just a little blood! Jaclyn was bleeding internally. He had already begun blood transfusions and was giving her platelets to help her blood clot. He told us he hoped she would begin to clot on her own over the next few hours. If not, he warned us that he might have to take her back to the operating room to fix the bleed. At the time I remember thinking that internal bleeding was our biggest nightmare. In reality, the surgeon was actually somewhat relieved that it was blood and not fluid retention around Jaclyn's heart. Bleeding was something the surgeon could fix. Jaclyn's heart not recovering from surgery would have been a much bigger problem. However, at the particular time this was happening, I saw blood oozing out of my child, and I didn't understand this difference. I was terrified!

    I immediately turned my anger toward the Fellow. The Fellow who let this continue for hours. The Fellow who ordered a chest x-ray at 10:30 pm and not another one later. The Fellow who had been doing ultrasounds of Jaclyn's neck but never of her heart! The Fellow who stood by while my daughter was bleeding internally.

    After the first hour of receiving blood and platelets, blood was still coming out of the tube inserted into Jaclyn's chest. A bag hung beside the bed, and we watched it fill. Initially it had 250 ml of Jaclyn's blood in it. After the first hour it was up to 400 ml of blood. The doctor wanted to wait another hour. But thirty minutes later, he came back to the room, looked at the bag that was continuing to fill with my daughter's blood, and he told us he could wait no longer. He said he would take her back to surgery. With a most serious look on his face, the face that in the past had always been so optimistic and calming to me, he said, "I will **fix** this." He expected to find a single vessel that had burst. He said, "It might take me forty-five minutes to an hour to find it, but once I do, it will take me about five minutes to fix it."

    While he was talking to us, he was writing on a piece of paper. He pushed the paper over the table for us to sign. It was a Consent for Surgery. As my husband signed the form, both of us became hysterical.

How could this be happening?

Because it was 9:00 am on a Sunday morning, the surgeon's staff members were not at the hospital. He had summoned his surgical nurses and his preferred anesthesiologist. An operating room had to be prepped. He told us it might be an hour before everything would be ready. Twenty minutes later he came back. Everything was ready. It was time.

We were escorted to the surgical waiting room in the main hospital. It was dark and locked. Only emergency surgeries occurred on Sunday mornings. Normally, volunteers manned the phones in the waiting room, receiving updates from the operating rooms and then relaying the information to the families. Not today. Instead, we were told to answer the phone ourselves, as it would be a nurse from the operating room telling us how things were going.

In addition to being scared beyond words, I also had intense guilt for not having prepared Jaclyn for this. Again, we didn't know she would require a ventilator again, let alone an emergency surgery. But I knew she would be angry for not being told.

An hour passed. No call from the operating room. We sat. We waited. We barely spoke. A little later the phone rang. A nurse said the surgeon was still working. It would take more time. Two and a half hours later we would see Jaclyn again. She had new steri-strips placed over the incision. The surgeon took great pains to go in through the same incision so Jaclyn would only have one chest scar. In fact, over the years, all four heart surgeries have been through the same incision. I can't say enough about the surgeon for this effort. While this emergency surgery wasn't open-heart, Jaclyn's chest was, again, re-opened. However, a new chest tube would have to be inserted and not in the same place as the old one. Another scar.

Each time Jaclyn faced surgery, Alan and I handled it differently. Over the years, while my husband worried that Jaclyn might not survive surgery, my brain refused to think that way. I could not come to grips with the notion that each surgery my daughter needed was life-threatening. I could not live with her on a day-to-day basis thinking that she could die. I wasn't lackadaisical in my understanding of the seriousness of her heart condition. In order to survive, I focused instead on the wonders of my Jaclyn. In the back of my mind, of course I knew the risks of her surgeries and the dangerous nature of what she was undergoing, but for self-preservation my mind didn't dwell on those things. Maybe I knew too much! I wasn't in denial. I was instead focusing on Jaclyn living…and nothing else. I couldn't control the outcome of her heart's recuperation and recovery each time she had surgery. One small thing I *could* do was at least ask about scarring and whether incisions could be made where old ones already existed. Sometimes this was possible, and other times it was not. But I had to ask. It was such a small thing I could do for my daughter, but to me it was the *only* thing I could do. Faced with little control over Jaclyn's well-being during these times, scar management became a focus of mine by default.

On that day, when the surgeon finally came out to say he had taken care of the bleeding, I almost knocked him over as I hugged him. He had expected to find a single vessel that had burst. That's not what he had found. Instead, there was generalized oozing and bleeding all over. He explained that if a person falls on the sidewalk and scrapes his/her arm, bleeding does not only occur from one place. Rather, oozing and bleeding come from the many areas of the skin that were scraped. He had to cauterize many, many such areas. That's what took so long.

We were told that one of the pain medications Jaclyn had started taking two days earlier could affect the platelets' ability to clot. This happens "in very rare cases," we heard. Although she had received that drug years ago after surgery without incident, this time it caused a problem. Again, an event that "barely ever" happens was now happening to Jaclyn.

But the surgeon fixed it. Another incision would need to heal, but at that time all that mattered was that this wonderful man had saved Jaclyn's life! She would come off the ventilator later the same day, without much turmoil. She had another chest tube. The first chest tube had just been removed, and now we were starting over again with a second. Jaclyn's color slowly returned to her skin. The huge amount of blood that had accumulated in her neck would have to be reabsorbed by the skin. "It might take days or weeks" we were told. The bruising was severe in her neck and upper chest, but at least that scare was behind us.

When Jaclyn began to awaken, we explained what had happened. I could hardly hold back my desire to have her talk. I was still worried about her brain. But she was sedated. As she awakened more, I waited for a cue. She began to speak—and she spoke and spoke and spoke. My fears were quietly put to rest, without anyone even knowing I had had them. What a relief!

We knew our surgeon ran his unit with a firm hand. We knew his word was final, and his demands on his staff were high. I wanted to have a talk with him about the Fellow. I wanted to know if the bleeding had been happening for hours. I could only surmise that the amount of blood coming out meant the bleeding was not short-lived. I wanted to know if the Fellow could have done more. But I never brought myself to ask. Whether the Fellow made a mistake or not, I will never know. What he actually said to her in private, I can only imagine. But suffice it to say, that particular Fellow never saw Jaclyn, or us, for the rest of our stay in the hospital.

On the first day of this hospitalization, we met Jenny, a nurse in PSHU who became Jaclyn's favorite. There were many nurses on The Unit who knew us from our repeated hospital stays over the years. But Jenny asked to be assigned to care for Jaclyn as often as she could. She enjoyed Jaclyn, and Jaclyn loved the attention. Jenny told us over and over how remarkable Jaclyn was, as she had seen many children and their families pass through the PSHU. Not only did we hear this from Jenny, but from other nurses and doctors too.

To brighten up Jaclyn's PSHU room, my mom had taken photographs of Ryan's and Joshua's faces and glued them atop traced, full-size drawings of their bodies. The boys colored each of their bodies and these hung on the wall in Jaclyn's PSHU room so she could see her brothers. In addition, my mom wrote inspirational sayings to Jaclyn and hung those on the wall too.

Ryan and Joshua visited Jaclyn in the hospital during the second week. Our pediatrician had to complete forms indicating that the boys were up-to-date with immunizations before they were allowed on the unit. They were nervous to see their sister in a hospital room with numerous machines. They were not used to fresh scars, multiple IVs, and her weakened state. They brought her bakery cookies and spent a bit of time watching movies with her. They missed her and needed to see her in-person to know she was okay.

Nurses and doctors saw our family a lot during hospitalizations—Alan and I were there around the clock, and my mom also stayed all day, every day. My in-laws visited and stayed with the boys at our house. My aunt and cousin were regular visitors too over the years, often bringing food to Alan and me, or staying with Jaclyn so we could run out to eat. While we often heard comments about how "exceptional" our family was, we simply wouldn't have managed those hospital stays any other way.

We went into the hospital for surgery with Jaclyn on March 13th. For no particular reason, Jaclyn wanted to be home by April 1st, April Fool's Day. At 11:00 pm, on March 31st, we were discharged. We made it home a few minutes shy of April Fool's Day. The boys had been sleeping at home that night with my aunt and uncle. They didn't know we were coming home. The next morning, they were surprised to be greeted by us. We had not told them Jaclyn was home. We told them to peek in her room. They found their sister sound asleep in her bed for the first time in twenty days. Two surgeries later—one planned and one definitely unplanned—she was home.

How Do You Thank Someone?

A few days after Jaclyn's emergency surgery, I was overcome with a need to thank our surgeon. For years he had performed surgeries on our daughter, as well as answered our many, many questions. In between surgeries, we would see him at an annual summer picnic held for families of children whose hearts had been repaired at his hospital. Each year, we stood in a long line with other grateful parents to have Jaclyn's picture taken with him, to shake his hand, and to thank him again for all he had done for our girl. And each year we were amazed at how many nurses and other doctors from PSHU continued to recognize us and remember our names. We had developed relationships with these doctors and nurses, and they continued showing their pleasure year after year when they'd see Jaclyn dancing at the picnic.

One year the hospital was to honor this surgeon and asked families to submit notes for a scrapbook. Jaclyn drew a picture, and I wrote him a thank you note. But this last time was different. The man had performed two surgeries on our daughter within a week, and she was okay! "Grateful" isn't a strong enough word to express our feelings for him. So after the second surgery scare was over, I crafted a poem that I framed and gave him. This is what I wrote:

How Do You Thank Someone?

Words don't exist to describe how we really feel
About the man who has made dreams for our child real.

How do you thank the person who has saved your daughter or son?
Gifts, hugs, and handshakes aren't enough; it simply can't be done.

It's a daunting task for us to extend our true gratitude
For your skill, patience, thoughtfulness and positive attitude.

When we brought Jaclyn to you almost ten years ago,
You answered all our questions as if you had no place else to go.

You told us on that first day that you would fix her heart,
With a look on your face indicating you meant it from the start.

You drew us pictures and diagrams, upside-down nonetheless,
With tremendous grace, patience, and ease that most truly did impress.

And when I asked to see, up close, your hands which held the key
To saving my Jaclyn's life, you didn't even balk at me.

You graciously extended your hands, across the table where we sat
You showed them, first palms up, then palms down,
and that was simply that.

It was something about your demeanor, about your hands,
about your face,
That made me believe my daughter wouldn't be to you just another case.

You demonstrated competence, but also compassion, concern and care.
And a doctor who empathizes that way is somewhat rare.

We will never forget how your treated Jaclyn after each surgery;
You stroked her back, smoothed her hair, and were as kind
as you could be.

You always take a moment to talk to Jaclyn during rounds.
We appreciate the time you spend; your energy knows no bounds!

Like so many other families, your hospital is far from our home,
But we come here for one reason, and for one reason alone.

That reason is you, Doctor Ilbawi, and the unit that you run.
We would follow you to the ends of the earth
because we cherish what you have done.

We could have taken Jaclyn for treatment to doctors anywhere,
But we've always felt that she was safe within your tender care.

So how do you thank someone who saves children's lives every day?
Telling him you appreciate him seems like such an insufficient way.

Maybe the highest compliment, the biggest honor we can bestow
Is believing in you and trusting you with the child we love so.

We hold a special place in *our* hearts and will forever be indebted to you.
Thank you for your skill and your kindness and keep doing what you do!

Lori, Alan, Jaclyn, Ryan and Joshua

Not Letting Anything Stand in Her Way

Jaclyn was ecstatic to be home from the hospital after two surgeries in less than three weeks. She was tired, sore, weak, bruised, and lighter in weight than when she went into the hospital, but she was just glad to be home. That first day she ate her favorite foods and went through the numerous cards and gifts that friends and family had sent to wish her a speedy recovery.

She wasn't ready to return to school; she needed to rebuild strength and general energy. During that first week home, the diligent student finished all missed school work. She would be out of school for five weeks, but the day she returned she was completely caught up. We were proud of that.

Jaclyn's pacemaker lead had been dislodged during the second emergency surgery—another hurdle to get through. We knew it would have to be replaced under her armpit via another surgery. But the doctors wanted her to heal first.

When Jaclyn came home, Ryan and Joshua were very protective of her. Alan and I had been away from them for most of twenty days, yet they came to understand that we did what we had to do. They were careful around her, though a bit perplexed that she couldn't walk up the stairs easily her first few days home or that she would fall asleep on the couch in the middle of her favorite shows and movies. They were patient when it was called for, and Jaclyn's healing continued at home.

One day during that first week, Jaclyn was sitting at the kitchen table eating lunch. One of her friends was on the baseball field at recess and noticed Jaclyn through our patio window. That child ran to the playground to inform all the fourth graders that Jaclyn was, indeed, home. About twenty children stood in a line, along the retaining wall in our backyard, waving and calling out to Jaclyn, welcoming her home. I had to help her out the patio door to sit outside and wave to her friends. With tears streaming down my cheeks, I videotaped that row of friends wishing my daughter a quick recovery. The school and Jaclyn's friends were amazing, and we were so very touched.

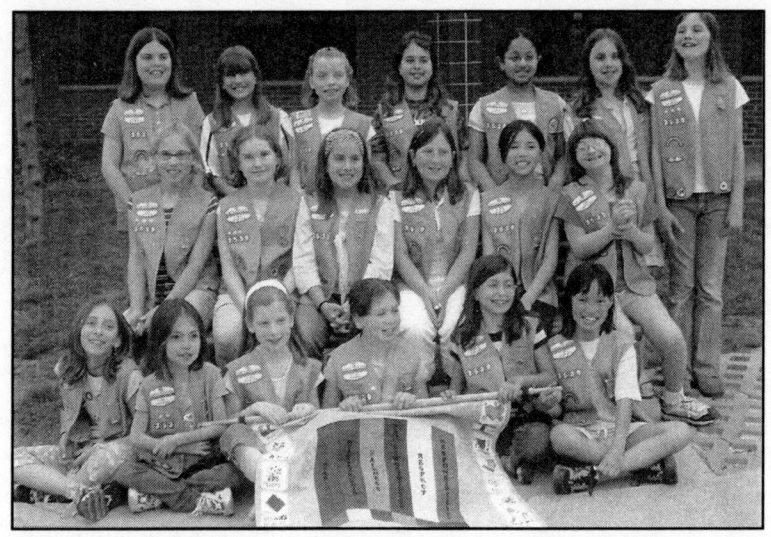

Jaclyn (second from left in the bottom row) and her Girl Scout Troup, Spring, 2006.

When Jaclyn returned to school, she was not allowed to climb steps, carry a backpack, or participate in gym or recess. Her friends made arrangements to ride the elevator with her in the school and to carry her backpack in and out of the building. Once again, they also took turns staying indoors at recess with her to keep her company.

It was early April, and the school talent show was scheduled for April 27th. Jaclyn desperately wanted to be in an act with her friends. But we realized she would not be able to perform their dance steps, as she had not been given the doctor's clearance to raise her arms over her breastbone. She was devastated. I told her I could choreograph a dance for her that she would be able to perform. She thought about it and decided she would do a solo. The song she chose was "Hit the

Road, Jack" by Ray Charles. I put together a two-minute dance for her, and she practiced and practiced.

Alan had mid-term exams for his MBA the weekend of the talent show and therefore missed it. I took the boys to the show and sat with a video camera in one hand and a digital camera in the other. My mom, aunt, uncle and cousin all came to watch too. I think there were about four hundred people in attendance. When Jaclyn saw the program for the evening show, she realized she was the only solo performance and got nervous. I reminded her that everybody would understand if she opted out of performing. She declined.

When it was time for her to go on, I sat in the audience spellbound. The music started. Jaclyn strutted out on the stage wearing black pants, a white sequined shirt, and silver sunglasses that were also covered in sequins. She had the sunglasses on her head. She walked to the middle of the stage and looked at me in the audience. I motioned to flip the sunglasses down onto her eyes because she had forgotten. Then she danced.

While taking both video and still photos at the same time, I was shaking and crying watching my daughter on that stage. I was crying at how proud I was of her. Ryan and Joshua were proud too. I was also emotional about how much she had been through and how courageous she was. She had just undergone two heart surgeries and had been home from the hospital only twenty-six days. In my head, I remembered a gaunt, bruised, sore, weak child in a hospital bed, asking the surgeon day after day when she could go home. Tubes, wires and machines had been hooked up to her for weeks. Emergency surgery had to be performed because she was bleeding internally. And there she was on stage, dancing through life! Nobody could have imagined what this child had been through. I cried so hard I could not hold the cameras still.

When Jaclyn's song ended, she strutted off stage. I hadn't realized that her fourth grade friends had been sitting behind me the whole time. Suddenly, I heard cheering like I had never heard before. I turned to see that she was getting a standing ovation. I couldn't contain myself.

Jaclyn came off the stage and walked to where her brothers and I were sitting. I gave her a quick high-five, smiled at her with immense pride, and watched her receive congratulatory remarks from the friends and peers that were surrounding her. I videotaped that too.

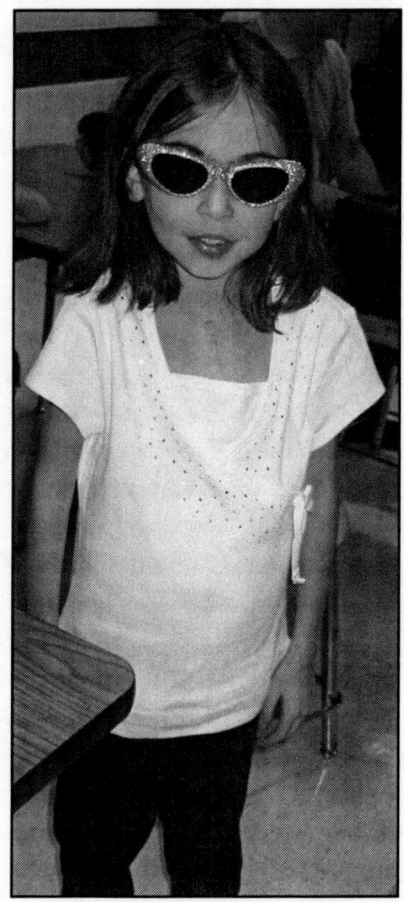

After her solo dance performance of "Hit the Road, Jack" at the school talent show, April, 2006.

Someone shouted out, "Good job!" Jaclyn scrunched her shoulders as if she's responding, "No big deal."

That night epitomized Jaclyn's life. She shone on that stage, after just having been through a fearful medical ordeal. But, as always, she didn't let it get in her way. Years later, people still remember Jaclyn's solo performance that night and tell all of us what an impression it made on them. It impressed us too.

Lessons Jaclyn Taught Me.

Persevere. No matter how bad things are, don't give up. Adapt if you have to. Make the best of things. Most of all, dance through life.

Dessert Fest

After Jaclyn's round of surgeries in the spring of 2006, we wanted to do something to thank the many people who had helped care for Ryan and Joshua and for those who had eased Jaclyn's recovery. We wanted to let them know how much we appreciated them and their friendship. Jaclyn turned ten on May 6th, and on May 7th we held an Open House Dessert Fest. Over 170 people came to our house to revel in the joy that Jaclyn had come through surgery well, to celebrate her 10th birthday, and to be thanked by us.

I baked, my mom baked, my aunt baked, and we bought a few desserts too. Various kinds of cakes, cookies, brownies, and dessert bars filled a huge table. We hired an entertainer to come and make balloon animals for the kids. It was a wonderful celebratory day. Jaclyn had made it through…again!

Two weeks after the Dessert Fest, Jaclyn had surgery to fix the dislodged pacemaker lead. She was going to miss all but one day of "Spirit Week" at school, the week that the whole student body dresses according to a theme. Jaclyn was very disappointed. With her teacher, she devised a plan to wear all the themes in the one day she would be there. That Monday morning, Jaclyn strutted into school, exuding her school spirit, with her crazy hair, Hawaiian lei, pajamas, hippie attire, and sports team paraphernalia all rolled into one outfit. She never let an experience pass her by.

On Tuesday she had surgery to change the pacemaker from a one-lead device to a two-lead device. Jaclyn had an incision under her armpit where the new pacemaker was inserted, and a second small incision on her stomach from the additional pacemaker lead. It was only one night in the hospital, but the recovery, again, forced her to wear a sling for six more weeks and not to lift her arm above her shoulder until the lead could more firmly implant in the heart wall. Between February and May, 2006, she had been through one ablation and four surgeries.

Acclimating to Hospital Life

Not only did we become familiar with hospitals over the years, but Jaclyn did too. I do not mean to say it ever got easier in the hospital, but rather that we got to know the ebb and flow of how things worked, which allowed us to have somewhat clear expectations. Because of many hospitalizations, lasting three to four weeks in duration, Jaclyn, Alan and I became somewhat like "experts" in hospital life. However, we still couldn't wait to be discharged so we could go home and be normal again.

Years ago, Tom Hanks was in a movie called *The Terminal*, about a foreigner who becomes trapped in an airport due to bureaucratic mix-ups and ends up living there. He learns the ropes regarding where to sleep, how to make money, and where to wash up, among other things, without being found out. Our lives in the hospital remind me of that movie.

For short one or two night hospital visits, there was less planning required. Even Jaclyn became hospital savvy for these short stays. She packed her own overnight bag: puzzle books, sharpened pencils, a chapter book, CDs, a CD player with headphones, extra batteries, DVDs, small board games, a hair brush, toothbrush, toothpaste, ponytail holders, socks, and underpants. She also remembered that her lips became dry and chapped in the hospital so she packed Chapstick. The only clothing needed was the outfit to wear home from the hospital. But even that outfit required some thought on her part. If she was to have a cardiac catheterization, she packed loose fitting pants because her groin area would be sore. If she was having surgery, she packed loose fitting shirts. Some procedures prohibited her from lifting her arms above her head for days, so shirts that buttoned up the front worked best under those conditions.

Jaclyn learned that there were many hours to fill while stuck in a hospital bed. She had determined which games she could play easily, especially with an IV in her arm, making her arm less usable. She packed only games with few pieces that could get lost.

Finally, Jaclyn packed her favorite things. When she was younger, she toted her favorite stuffed animals to the hospital—Puppy, Callie Kitty, and So-So Kitty—plus her pastel green and blue blanket. As she got older, the choice of stuffed animals changed, but the same thinning and worn blanket continued to accompany us on all hospital stays. She knew she did not like hospital food so she packed her own snacks too.

However, when a lengthier hospital stay would be required, we shifted into a different way of living. While Jaclyn packed more games and movies, for the most part her packing was similar for short and long hospitalizations. For Alan and me, long hospital stays were a whole new ballgame. We packed many days worth of clothes and kept them in a suitcase in the trunk of our car. We also stored a laundry bag in the trunk that was parked in the hospital lot. In Jaclyn's PSHU or ICU room, we kept an overnight bag, containing only toiletries and clothes for the next day. We would go to the car to exchange the dirty clothes for clean ones daily.

We also packed lots of reading materials because there were countless hours to sit and wait. Not only was the day of surgery usually a very long one, but subsequent days after surgery were also times that Jaclyn would be sedated and sleeping. A way to pass the time was to read—newspapers and news magazines that didn't require a lot of my attention worked well. As Jaclyn would begin to wake, I'd often read chapter books aloud to her.

Our packing list also contained other essential items. We would bring our phone book and Alan's laptop computer which we used as a means to update friends, family, and neighbors about Jaclyn's progress. It was tiring to repeat progress reports about Jaclyn's condition over and over again. Before anyone had e-mail, we used to leave updates on our outgoing voice mail message at home. Friends and family members would call our phone to hear progress reports. But once e-mail became widespread, we simply sent updates to a master list of people every few days. This mode of communication was much easier.

In addition to these items, we also packed snacks to avoid having to buy all our food from cafeterias or vending machines. We brought our own soap and towels, because hospital ones are rough. And it became my responsibility to pack our good luck charms as well. While I'm not the kind of person who normally believes in those things, during Jaclyn's hospitalizations, I did bring the old standby items that had been with us through each surgery and each procedure.

For instance, when Jaclyn was an infant, she loved the Disney movie *101 Dalmations*. She had a pair of red and white Dalmation socks that said "One tough pup" on them. She wore them to her first cardiac catheterization, the day they told us fixing her heart was "doable." She wore them to her first surgery (at age six weeks) and second surgery (at six months). By her third surgery, at age three, the socks no longer fit. Yet they were a good luck charm, and we needed a new pair.

My mother was on a mission to find a bigger pair of the same socks. With my aunt's help, they called every Disney Store they could find. Nobody had the socks. My mother called Disney headquarters and explained the situation—that Jaclyn had worn the socks through her first two surgeries, that they were good luck, and that she had to have a bigger pair for her next surgery. The Customer Service Representative took up the cause and decided that if he had to look through every box in the warehouse to find them, he would. Days later, three pairs of Dalmation socks appeared in my mother's mailbox—at no charge. By age nine, Jaclyn had the idea to put the socks, which were again too small for her, on one of the stuffed animals that came with us to the hospital. Brilliant!

"Day" versus "Night" was never of grave concern to hospital staff. Patients, even children, are examined, throughout all hours of the day and night while in the hospital. Jaclyn's vital signs were taken every two to four hours. She was examined by nurses and/or residents as they perused the PSHU or ICU floor—often occurring at all hours. Respiratory therapists came into her room to check the status of ventilators and oxygen throughout the day and night. Chest x-rays were taken each morning, between 4:00 am and 5:00 am, so results would be ready for viewing by doctors during morning rounds. There was no good time to sleep in a PSHU or ICU room. Children tended to get their days and nights confused, as they were awakened so often during the night. Consequently, Jaclyn slept a lot during daylight hours. We stayed with her each night until she was asleep, so our sleep was disturbed as well.

Doctors' rounds were an important part of each day at the hospital. Often, this was the only chance parents had to see the surgeon or cardiologist. This was the time to ask questions, get progress reports, and find out what needed to happen before Jaclyn could be discharged. We were always in her room for rounds, unless we were asked to leave due to an emergency on the unit or because it was time for nurses' shift change. On surgery days, rounds tended to be around 7:30 am. On non-surgery days, rounds were later and the times varied. Weekends were our least favorite times to be in the hospital, because doctors were often more scarce. Attending physicians were available, but this was not the same as seeing the doctor who knew your child the best. Rounds sometimes did not occur until noon or even later on weekends.

When we couldn't get a room in the Guest House across the street from the hospital, or years later when the Guest House was no longer in existence, we adapted our sleeping arrangements. Parents were not encouraged to sleep in PSHU or ICU with their child. Many of the children having cardiac surgeries tended to be infants or toddlers. It was actually easier to slip out and sleep on a couch down the hall, or even at a hotel when the child was a baby. Many parents did this. But when Jaclyn was older and could verbalize her feelings, leaving her was almost impossible.

At older ages, Jaclyn wanted one of us in her room all the time. We wanted to be there too. This meant one of us could sleep on a chair in the family waiting room, if one was available. The other one of us would attempt to sleep in her room on a chair that semi-reclined. These chairs were a definite deterrent to sleeping, which we imagine is one reason most parents don't stay.

"Sleeping" in PSHU or ICU with your child is really an impossibility. There is really no "sleep" to be had. Patients are awakened throughout the night for various exams and monitors beep incessantly at all hours. Alarms beep when signals are not being picked up, when a child rolls onto a lead, and, in Jaclyn's case, when her heart rate and oxygen levels fluctuated. When her numbers dropped, even momentarily, alarms sounded.

Also, IV pumps beeped after they finished administering medications and/or maintenance fluids. These machines beeped until someone turned them off. This environment was not conducive to rest. While Jaclyn would doze throughout daylight hours to make up for lack of sleep at night, we, as parents, didn't have that luxury. After years of being in hospital rooms with Jaclyn, Alan and I learned how to read the various machines and monitors that were hooked up to our daughter. We knew when a pump was beeping due to being empty versus having erred. Nurses didn't always respond quickly to machines that were empty because they were caring for multiple patients at the same time. But when Jaclyn would just fall asleep after countless hours of wakefulness, ringing alarms woke her. Alan and I got brazen by the fourth or fifth hospitalization and muted the alarms on occasion when we knew they were simply making noise because they were empty. The alarms still sounded at the nurses' station down the hall from PSHU to alert nurses that they were empty, but at least the sound was muted next to Jaclyn's ear. We only did this when Jaclyn was trying desperately to sleep. However, we received a lecture from nurses asking us to refrain from touching the machines. We certainly wouldn't have endangered our child—we just wanted peace so she could rest. We understood the reason for the request and never intervened again.

But through it all, Jaclyn did not let a hospital bed stand in her way of having some fun. She packed games from home to play. We watched funny movies, cartoons, and Broadway musicals. She brought CDs and often could be heard down the hall belting out the words to her favorite songs. Doctors, nurses, and other specialists often poked their heads into her PSHU room to see the little girl, with dark brown hair in ponytails and big eyes, who was not deterred by procedures or even surgery. When Jaclyn broke into songs from her favorite musical, *Wicked*, her doorway was often packed with people who could not believe what they were seeing or hearing. Despite monitors and IVs attached to her, medications being pumped into her, and bruises and scars to heal, she would entertain herself and often the surgical staff as well.

Lessons Jaclyn Taught Me.

There's never a bad time for having fun. Even when feeling lousy, sore, and tired, Jaclyn managed to ask, "Can we play a game?" Games and music can help people feel better. Try it. A good attitude definitely matters.

Sleeping and Eating at the Hospital

Sleep, or lack thereof, was definitely an issue for Jaclyn and us when she was hospitalized. Showering at the hospital was another story. After the Guest House's demise and prior to the opening of the Ronald McDonald House, we no longer had a clean, private place to shower each day. We often used the tub room on the rehabilitation floor of the hospital.

Eating was often logistically difficult when Jaclyn was hospitalized too. Hospital cafeterias got tiring after eating so many meals in them for so many weeks at a time, but they sufficed. We were also lucky to have family members run to restaurants to bring us food or to stay with Jaclyn while we took a break from the tedium of PSHU. When nurses had meals delivered, Alan and I often placed our own orders with theirs. We adapted the best we could.

A tray of donuts was delivered each morning to the ICU family waiting room. These donuts sat on a table throughout much of the day. During Jaclyn's most recent surgery, I remember sitting on a recliner in the waiting room, still wearing the sweatpants and t-shirt I had slept in the previous night. I had not yet showered because the facilities were being used, when a perky mom struck up a conversation with me. After another rough night with Jaclyn, I was not up for a friendly chat. Nor did I look as well dressed as this woman.

Nevertheless, she initiated a conversation by saying, "Don't they know Moms don't *eat* this kind of stuff?" Since I had personally consumed at least a dozen of those donuts during our twenty-day stay, I wasn't the appropriate one for her to be asking. Those donuts were often my only sustenance on days that weren't going well, making a run to the cafeteria impossible. This woman asked if my child had been at the hospital long. When I told her we were closing in on three weeks, she was quite surprised. Then I heard that her son came in to the emergency room the night before due to a peanut allergy. She was concerned that he was missing soccer practice that day. I sat in my sweats, with my mussed up hair, tired and in need of a shower, but not wanting to leave the unit until after rounds. It was at that moment that I realized she would never be able to live the way I had been living in that hospital. Later that afternoon, I saw her son leaving ICU—discharged less than twenty-four hours after arriving. She had made it through one night in ICU. I ate another donut.

While I realize that hospitals are in business to care for sick patients, not families, I do believe that family members' needs should be taken into account. After all, families are the ones having to care for these children and patients once they are discharged. I understand that parents and families can be somewhat of a nuisance to hospital staff with a multitude of questions and requests. I also believe, at the same time, that it is beneficial that families be present, if possible. Parents and families help the patients, not just physically by handling some of their child's needs, but also psychologically simply by their loving presence. Our hospital has now built a Ronald McDonald House where patients' families can stay. This should be an improvement over what we have sometimes endured over the years.

A Hospital is a Very Sad Place

When Jaclyn had her open-heart surgery (and emergency surgery) at age 9 ½ , she was in the hospital for twenty days. In addition to her PSHU room, the family waiting room became our home-away-from-home. This was where parents sat, sometimes slept, used the telephone or the computer, ate, watched television, used the bathroom, and waited. Parents were not allowed to be on the unit when nurses changed shifts—at 7:00 am, 3:00 pm, and 11:00 pm every day. Each shift change took about an hour. The family waiting room was the place to wait when not with your child.

Many families shared this waiting room. It was a place where parents often chatted with each other; we heard a lot of stories in that room. There was a sort of bonding relationship that sometimes occurred among families. Some of the stories were about children with pneumonia or RSV. These families stayed only a few days. It was heartbreaking to learn of the family whose little boy had a brain tumor, or the toddler who choked on a hot dog and was brain-damaged, or the family whose teenage son had a tumor on his spine and the doctors didn't know if he would walk once the tumor was removed.

When Jaclyn was three and having her second open-heart surgery, one other family was in the waiting room with us day after day. Other parents came and went, but this family was there around the clock, as we were. We learned that their daughter also had open-heart surgery, and we spent countless days chatting, catching up on each day's experiences, and sharing our concerns. When she was discharged, before Jaclyn, we were so happy for them! Years later, I still remember that the girls' name was Grace, and I hope she's okay.

During Jaclyn's most recent surgery, we met a lot of families. It started when I asked a mom if her son had a good day. Then she asked about Jaclyn. We would talk over days about how even small steps forward were encouraging. One night, her son was having a terrible time. While we were in Jaclyn's ICU room, we could see many doctors and nurses congregating in his room, only a few doors down. The hustle and bustle in and out of that room was frightening. Later when we saw the parents, we didn't know what to say. I remember having a sick-to-my-stomach-feeling. Not knowing what was happening was hard, but due to confidentiality, nurses were not able to let us know how he was. We only wanted the little boy, who we had never met, to be all right. We had a sort of camaraderie with his family, from our shared experience of having a sick child. The next day, when I saw the mom, she told me he was doing better. She explained that if he had another "crash" like that, they didn't know if he'd make it. I cried, tears of fear, but also tears of happiness that it was behind them.

There is this feeling I often had when in the hospital with Jaclyn, a feeling that is hard to describe. It was not difficult to discern when another child in PSHU was not doing well. There would often be a lot of doctors and nurses coming and going. Sometimes we were even asked to leave the unit while there was a crisis in another room. Fortunately, this did not happen too often, but it was very troubling when it did occur.

When another child was having difficulties, I have experienced a feeling over which I am ashamed. The only way to describe it is to call it an "I'm-so-glad-it's-not-happening-to-us" feeling. Of course I wished for all the children to recover quickly and be well. But at the same time, I had been so afraid of Jaclyn having a crisis from which she couldn't recover that I have had momentary feelings of relief when the crisis was another child's and not my own. I am embarrassed by this emotion, however real it is.

During the most recent hospitalization, one night Alan had gone to "make our beds" down the hall on the pull-out chairs. It was almost 10:00 pm, and a man was already in that room. Alan asked if he had been planning to spend the night, in which case we would have had to find other sleeping arrangements. The man said,

"No, we're just waiting for our daughter to pass away. Then we'll be leaving." Terribly upset, my husband told the man he was sorry and proceeded to leave the room. When he returned to Jaclyn's room, he was pale and speechless. He didn't want to tell me in front of Jaclyn what had transpired. Later he informed me that a family was waiting for their child to die. I didn't even know this family, but I got sick in the bathroom. I couldn't sleep. I was traumatized.

The next morning I had a lump in my throat. I looked at my Jaclyn, my child who had made it through so much, and I was eternally grateful. My mind wandered to a family I did not even know. I kept thinking of how awful it must have been for that father to utter the words he did to my husband. I imagined that, on this day, a family was spending their day childless, that their daughter had died. I could not fathom the pain of that experience.

Later that day, Jaclyn took her first steps out of her ICU room. She had been in the hospital for eighteen days so far and was finally strong enough to walk. With an IV pole in tow, she strutted down the hallway, albeit slowly and weakly. As she walked past all the PSHU rooms, Alan saw that father again. His child was all right. I cried, but at the same time, I smiled because my daughter finally had enough strength to walk.

The range of feelings I experienced during hospitalizations ran the gamut. I felt hope for children on the unit to get better. I felt jealous when other children were discharged while Jaclyn stayed. I also felt grateful that my child came home after each surgery, even though sometimes we felt like we would never get out of there. While I know intuitively that hospitals are places where lives are mostly saved, to me they still represent tremendous sadness and fear.

Lessons Jaclyn Taught Me.

Relish little things. A good day in the hospital might mean that Jaclyn was able to eat or drink something and keep it down. Or a good day could be defined as her having enough energy to watch a few cartoons. Good days were sometimes short-lived, but Jaclyn tried to make the most of them, whether that meant playing a few games of Gin Rummy or listening to a few favorite songs or working for a few minutes on a Lite Bright design.

The Things They Don't Tell You

When you have a chronically ill child, there is a lot of information to take in. There is initial shock, disbelief, depression, anger, and a barrage of other emotions. There is also the diagnosis which must be comprehended, at some level, by the family. We have learned that families seem to handle learning about the diagnosis differently. Our way has always been to simply gather as much information as we could. We asked countless questions to each and every doctor who treated our daughter. I believe we were fairly medically savvy in regards to Jaclyn's condition, even though neither of us have direct medical training. We learned what to look for regarding clinical symptoms or behavioral changes in Jaclyn. We really knew a lot about our child's health.

Some families that we have encountered who also live with chronic illness seem to ask fewer questions. Perhaps they don't ask the kinds of questions we ask because of language barriers. Perhaps they simply do not want to know the details that we feel are our right to know. Another possibility is that both my husband and I are with Jaclyn for the duration of her stay so we can actually see the doctors, surgeons, cardiologists, residents, interns, nurses, and respiratory therapists who cared for her. We had access to these people on a daily basis, and we were not shy about asking questions. We learned from these various professionals more about Jaclyn's heart condition, what was "normal" given her anatomy, and what was clinically problematic.

I believe this helped us give Jaclyn the best care we could have, over the long-run.

We have also been fortunate to have insurance covering Jaclyn's medical treatment; Alan works for a company with fabulous benefits. When Jaclyn was two years old, we started to get concerned that her lifetime maximum insurance benefit would be reached in a matter of years, because of the expense of all the surgeries and hospitalizations. Alan began to work with the benefits department at his company to see if the lifetime maximum could be lifted. More than a year later, he received an email from a manager stating that Jaclyn's case was the inspiration behind the removal of the lifetime benefit maximum. Back then, unlimited health insurance was relatively unheard of. Alan was also able to take sick days/personal days/vacation days that allowed him to be with our daughter, even for extended hospitalizations. These benefits have allowed both of us, as parents, to be with Jaclyn night and day. This is not the case for some of the children we have seen in ICU or PSHU. Having a child with chronic illness can bear a tremendous burden for a family—financially and emotionally—and everyone handles it in their own way.

Lessons Jaclyn Taught Me.

There is no right way to handle illness and/or hospitalizations. Some days, especially right after surgery, Jaclyn would simply sleep while her recovery began. Other days she could tolerate only movies, music, or having books read to her. As her recovery would progress, she would dictate an activity level that often included making crafts, or playing game after game to pass the time—all in her hospital bed. We heard from many health care professionals that Jaclyn's style was unique. Nurses and doctors told us they were not accustomed to PSHU rooms being inundated with games, books, DVDs and CDs, but this was simply how we handled hospital stays. Other families passed the days in different ways, but Jaclyn insisted on being busy when she was able.

How Do You Do It?

Many people over the years have told Jaclyn how brave she was to get through this procedure or that surgery. Alan and I have certainly fielded our share of questions asking how we did it too. The answer is simple. It's actually one of the easiest questions I can answer about caring for Jaclyn: We did what we had to do. We didn't stop and think about it. We didn't just decide one day to do it. Sometimes people are thrust into circumstances that they don't expect, that they didn't ask for, that they didn't plan for, that aren't even fair. But we dealt with it as best as we could *because we had no choice.*

Over the years, we have done whatever was required for our child to be okay. We got second opinions by having Jaclyn's EKGs, echocardiograms and surgical notes sent to other doctors. We even took her to other states to see different doctors. She went through years of therapies: speech therapy to eventually learn how to eat, physical therapy to work on strength and endurance, occupational therapy to address fine-motor skills, and occasional behavior therapy to deal with her eating issues. As parents of a chronically ill child, we didn't have time to stop and wonder how to get through something. We just did it.

While in the hospital with Jaclyn, life was not normal by any stretch of the imagination. In her first three years, Jaclyn was hospitalized over one hundred days for various procedures, surgeries and illnesses. It was a tough road. Looking back, I am sometimes amazed at the realization that Alan and I survived those days. But we did. We had each other and great support from family and friends too. As Jaclyn got older, her open-heart surgeries were brutal. Recoveries were tremendously difficult. By then we knew too much. I'm not sure if that made it better or worse.

However, outside of the hospital, our life and Jaclyn's life were normal. Sure, "normal" for Jaclyn meant medications, therapies, medical equipment, numerous doctor appointments, and occasional challenges, but that was just the way her life was and we lived it day to day without much thought about it as being difficult. For us it wasn't difficult; it was just how it needed to be.

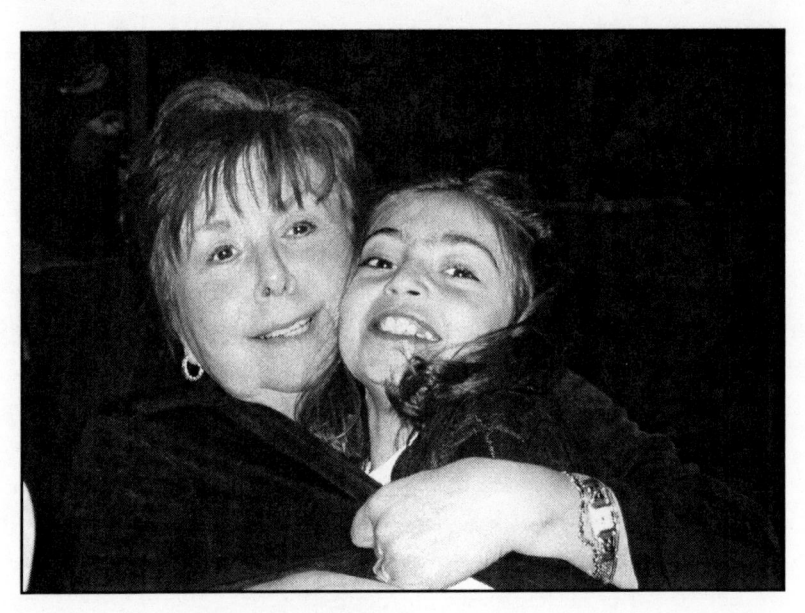

Mema and Jaclyn hugging, June, 2006.

One of the things we were most proud of in our handling of Jaclyn's health has been our insistence not to think of her, or to have others think of her, as a "sick child." And more importantly, Jaclyn never thought of herself as sick either. She knew her heart didn't grow the way it was supposed to grow. She knew it required surgical repair. But she did not think of herself as different from any of her friends. She did not question why this happened to her. She did not get angry

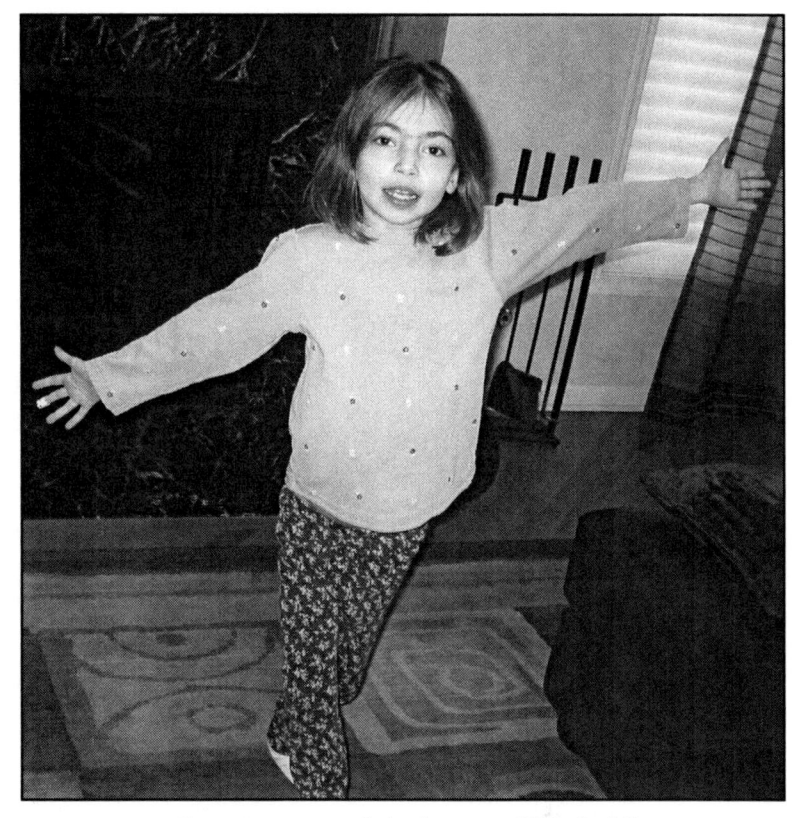

Dancing around the house to "Wicked."

about it. She did not act out over it, though she certainly had a right to. She dealt with it as just part of who she was. She required many doctors' appointments. She had procedures and surgeries. She took medicine. She slept with oxygen often. She was small and petite. But she didn't let her medical history get in the way of her life!

We, as a family, didn't let Jaclyn's heart condition define our lives either. When she was younger and needed medical equipment, we took it with us. It was more difficult to travel then, but we did it. When she was older, we continued to live our lives and not let her condition slow us down. We always had activities planned. Jaclyn was engaged in various endeavors, both in and outside of school. When she wasn't in the hospital, which was most of the time, our family did things and went places regularly.

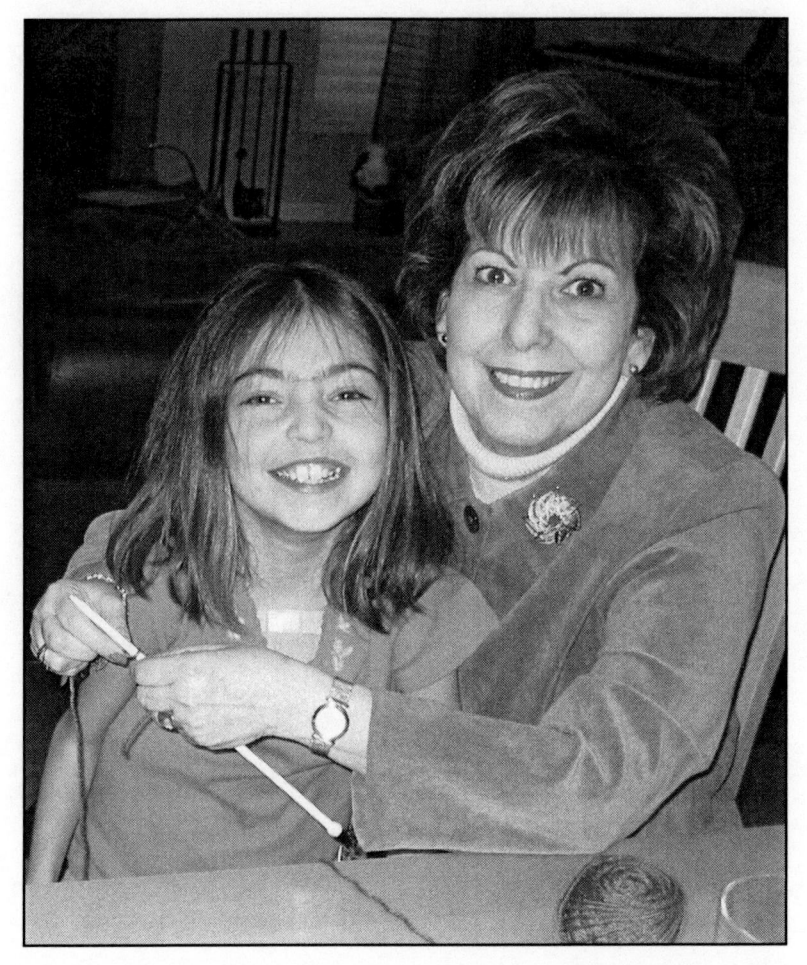

Learning how to knit with Aunt Ellen, April, 2006.

We took many family trips too. Initially, I feared that Jaclyn would get sick while we were away and we wouldn't be near our cardiologist. But the choice was to either never leave town or to give it a try and tackle the problem of finding a doctor on vacation if she got sick. The first time we took a trip, I insisted that our cardiologist recommend a doctor in the city where we were going, just to be safe. In all our travels, Jaclyn only needed to see a doctor one time; he called our cardiologist at home to confer, but everything was fine. We consciously tried not to allow Jaclyn's heart condition to limit what we could do. When she required medical intervention, she got it—we'd be in medical mode. But on a day-to-day basis, nobody could tell by looking at Jaclyn, or by seeing how she acted or how we treated her, that she was anything other than a healthy child. Our determination to give Jaclyn, and our family, a regular life helped enable us to carry on in spite of the adversity we faced. This is something I am particularly proud of in our handling of Jaclyn and her medical condition over the years.

Lessons Jaclyn Taught Me.

A child deserves a life full of fun, humor, good times and memories. Many families who live with illness are so mentally and physically consumed by it that they are overwhelmed by the idea of engaging in "regular" family life. Jaclyn taught me, and our family, that her heart didn't have to be the first thing on our minds every day and every night. While extra attention to medications *was* necessary on a daily basis, that alone didn't stop this child from demanding as "normal" a childhood as her brothers had.

The Best Summer Ever

During the first half of 2006, Jaclyn endured one ablation, the addition of a pacemaker, and four surgeries. Then she danced in the school talent show! That was our girl. Nothing stood in her way. In May she had her tenth birthday, and we threw the Open House Dessert Fest to thank everyone for all their help during her surgeries and recoveries.

Summer of 2006 was her best summer ever. Despite beginning the season with her arm in a sling, due to surgery to replace the pacemaker lead, she did not slow down. She finished fourth grade and dove into summer vacation head-on. Because of her recent scars, she was supposed to be out of the sun. Just as a suntan can darken skin, it can also darken scars, but the darkened red color would be permanent.

Jaclyn's scars had always lightened enough to have blended into her skin almost completely. The older she got, the more aware I was of continuing to care for her scars as best as I could. When Jaclyn was six weeks old, after her first surgery, we were told that scars should be out of the sun for a whole year. That wasn't a problem when she was younger. But at age nine and then ten, it was harder to stay out of sun when it was hot, when there was recess, when friends played outside, and when the summer pool opened. I slathered her skin and scars with the highest protective sunscreen I could find. But that wasn't enough. Instead of wearing normal, sleeveless shirts in the summer,

Jaclyn often wore "rash guard" shirts everywhere she went because they had UV protection built into them and they covered her armpit and her chest scar. She hated them, but she wore them.

At the beginning of the summer, we engaged in a lot of indoor activities just to avoid the sun's rays. Jaclyn wasn't able to raise her arm above her shoulder until the Fourth of July. She was disappointed not to be allowed to go to the pool. Instead, the kids swam in a backyard blow-up pool. My mom bought us a canopy that we placed over the pool, to keep Jaclyn out of the sun. We invited friends over a lot for games and movies. We went to the arcade, the library, to lunch, and just spent a lot of quality time at home early that summer. Watching *The Price is Right, Who Wants to Be a Millionaire?* and *Family Feud* were often the highlights of Jaclyn's morning. She really enjoyed game shows. We played a lot under the patio umbrella, in the shade. And the three kids found a new favorite outdoor activity—pushing each other on the hammock. As the sun would travel across the sky throughout the day, the boys and I would move the hammock around the yard to keep it as shaded as possible. Jaclyn, as always, blasted music through the backyard speakers whenever we were outside.

By late June, I decided to take the kids to visit a girlfriend and her family in Cleveland. Alan was travelling internationally for two weeks for his MBA. So the kids and I hit the road for our first car trip. When we arrived, Jaclyn presented my friends' daughters with a tie-dye kit and a bunch of plain, white undershirts. The five kids began to make tie-dye shirts the moment we arrived. We had a fantastic time.

For the rest of the summer, once Jaclyn was cleared to raise her arm, we spent a lot of time at the local pool. Wearing rash guards, Jaclyn stayed in shallow water, and she really worked hard on her swimming. She often brought pool toys so that when her friends wanted to swim in deeper water, she could stand on the side of the pool and throw toys to them. At least this way she could still play with them.

The Heart Institute Picnic was fun for Jaclyn too, because it would be a time for her to see Jenny, her favorite nurse. This was the picnic the hospital hosted each year for families of children whose hearts had been repaired by our surgeon. Each time we had gone back to the hospital for post-surgery check-ups, Jaclyn would beg me to take her to the PSHU to see if Jenny was there. Often, she wasn't on call those days. But they e-mailed each other throughout the summer, hoping to find a day to get together for a visit. The picnic turned out to be it. At the event, Jaclyn saw all the nurses, doctors and, of course, our surgeon. Many comments were made about how healthy she looked, coming from the people who had witnessed the horrors of those days in PSHU. But what I recall the most from that day was the sight of Jaclyn and Jenny dancing the afternoon away as the DJ played song after song—many at Jaclyn's request. Jaclyn led the congo line, danced the limbo, and hula hooped in a contest that day.

In July, Jaclyn suddenly unbuckled her own car seat. Because she was small and light, she still sat in a front-harness car seat. But due to lack of strength and/or feeling in her fingertips, she was not able to push the plastic releases together to unlatch the buckle. She was ten years old and still unable to get out of her own car seat. But one day, she just did it. It might sound like a trivial accomplishment, but to us it was monumental. We didn't care how it actually transpired; we just celebrated the moment with her.

Later that summer, she was finally able to snap and unsnap buttons on pants. She had been wearing elastic pants, shorts, skirts or dresses her whole life because she couldn't fasten regular pants. So once she mastered this task, we went on a shopping spree to finally buy regular pants. She was so excited! Again, these may seem like trivial successes, but to Jaclyn and to us, they represented definite progress!

Jaclyn also tried riding her bike more often during the summer. She was hoping to gain enough strength in order to peddle fast and balance without training wheels. She was practicing a lot—something she had previously shied away from. And when we got a basketball hoop installed in our driveway, it was Jaclyn, as much as Ryan and Joshua, who went outside to practice shooting hoops. She was so proud when she'd make a basket. "Yes!" she'd shout.

Toward the middle of the summer, our family headed to the Wisconsin Dells to the water parks. With doctor's approval, we all climbed over 100 steps to reach the top of the water slides and careen down on inner tubes. Even Jaclyn did this—over and over and over again. She wasn't deterred by the heat, the exhausting steps, or the long lines. We had a ball.

The summer was filled with lots of laughter, tons of family time, thousands of games, girlfriends sleeping over, and voracious amounts of reading on Jaclyn's part. Jaclyn really matured a lot during that summer too.

Alan had a second international trip in August, 2006, again for his MBA. Seeing how well Jaclyn had recovered, and sensing that Alan and I could really use some time together after the year of surgeries and hospitalizations, my mom volunteered to stay with our kids so I could meet Alan in London and Paris for a week. But the day before I was to fly to meet him, terrorists were stopped before they could attack flights in London. My mom wouldn't let me go on the trip so I, along with many other MBA candidate spouses who were to travel abroad, cancelled our trips. Because of the many cancelled flights in London, it took Alan four days to get a flight home to Chicago.

He arrived home on Monday. Tuesday the five of us spent the day at the local pool. It was a beautiful day. I grilled Jaclyn's favorite steaks for dinner that night. My mom felt badly that we weren't in Europe, so she encouraged Alan and me to go away for a few days. We found a Bed and Breakfast in Michigan where we could go for two nights. My mom and cousin had planned to take the kids to an amusement park on Wednesday. At bedtime, Jaclyn told us she probably wouldn't sleep well that night because she was so excited about the amusement park. She couldn't wait!

One Day

  Wednesday, August 16th, we walked to school to see the class postings for the new school year. It was seven days before fifth grade was to begin, and Jaclyn was anxious to see who her teacher would be and whether Bethany, her best friend, would be in her class. When she saw that they would not be together, Jaclyn was noticeably upset. Walking home, I reminded her that she and Bethany would still have lunch and recess together and that being in different classes did not mean they wouldn't still be best friends. She held back her tears of disappointment.

  When we got home, my mom and cousin were in the driveway, ready for their fun day at the amusement park. Alan and I were also ready to go to Michigan for two nights, a highly anticipated respite for us to be alone together. We kissed the kids goodbye and told them to have fun. Jaclyn ran up to me, put her arms around my waist and wrapped her feet around my legs for a "bear hug," almost knocking me over in the process. We loaded Jaclyn, Ryan, and Joshua into my cousin's car and waved as they drove off, excitedly, to the amusement park. I ran upstairs to put cards under each of their pillows. When I had thought I was going to Europe for a week, I had bought each of them a greeting card saying I missed them, that I'd see them soon, to have fun and to behave for their grandmother. Jaclyn loved getting greeting cards. I placed the cards under their pillows for them to find when they arrived home from the amusement park.

Alan and I drove to Michigan and spent the day wandering around the lake and quaint town. Before dinner, we were sitting on a rocker at our Bed and Breakfast, enjoying the peace and quiet. It was Alan's idea to call the kids to see how their day was going. I had planned to call them later at night when they might be home, not while they were still at the amusement park. But he insisted. He dialed my cousin's cell phone, spoke briefly, then grabbed my hand and pulled me into the Bed and Breakfast. All I recall him saying was that Jaclyn fell, and we had to go. We threw our clothes into our suitcase and ran out, as my husband yelled to the host of the Bed and Breakfast that we had to leave for an emergency. We had been in Michigan for only a few hours. It was sometime around 6:00 pm.

Once we got out of town and onto the main highway, it occurred to me that Jaclyn might have broken a bone if she had indeed fallen. I remember my husband saying something about her falling and not breathing. I assumed that meant she might have had the wind knocked out of her. That's as far as my brain went with that information. I recall being rather calm in the car, as I felt confident that my mom could handle something as simple as a fall, even if it meant a broken bone. The fact that Jaclyn was not breathing never figured into my thinking.

It occurred to me that if Jaclyn was being taken to a hospital, perhaps I should call the staff to inform them that the medical history my mom undoubtedly relayed shouldn't concern them. After all, my daughter was fine, I reasoned. So while Alan drove like a maniac towards Chicago, I calmly called the hospital. I remember saying that my daughter was either en route to the hospital, or perhaps already there. I told the person who answered the phone that I was calling simply to fill in the blanks about Jaclyn's medical history or medications in case they were alarmed. I was put on hold.

Many moments later, a nurse came to the phone. I was expecting to be told that Jaclyn broke her arm when she fell and that she needed a cast. That was it. In my mind, all I could think about was *another sling, another bump in the road. One more thing to recover from. Poor Jaclyn.*

The nurse began speaking in a monotone voice, very matter-of-factly. This is what she said: "Your daughter was running. She fell. She wasn't breathing. People nearby tried to revive her. Paramedics were called. They tried to revive her. They shocked her. They prepared her for transport and continued trying to revive her. They couldn't. She died." Then the nurse paused. I was silent.

My husband kept asking me what the nurse was saying. I didn't answer him, as he continued speeding on the highway. I finally yelled at the nurse on the phone, "I DON'T KNOW WHO YOU'RE TALKING ABOUT! I'm calling about my daughter, Jaclyn Silberman. S-I-L-B, as in boy, E-R-M-A-N." Then I said something like, "my daughter fell, she might have a broken bone. SILBERMAN." Alan was yelling at me to tell him what the nurse had said about Jaclyn. I waved him off and told the nurse I wanted to speak to my mother. I assumed my mom would get on the phone and tell me Jaclyn had broken a bone, but that she was fine.

It took a long time for my mom to get to the phone. I was waiting for her regular voice. Instead, I could barely hear her. She muttered these words to me, almost inaudibly: "just get here." I dropped the cell phone on the floor of the front seat of the car. I stared at my husband who was driving like a crazy person. My hands were holding the sides of my face. I sat in silence, unable to speak, move, think, breathe. Alan kept asking me, over and over, how Jaclyn was. Finally, I told him what the nurse had said. I repeated her story. And when I got to the end of what she relayed to me, I said, "and she told me Jaclyn died." He screamed, "Nooooo!" But I wasn't crying. I might have started shaking by then, but I refused to take in what I had just heard a nurse say to me. Maybe this is what it means to be in shock.

I don't remember much from that car ride. At some point I told Alan we needed a helicopter. I said that there had to be someone we could call to arrange a helicopter to fly us to the hospital. We were about four hours away, and because it was rush-hour, we did not know how long it would take to get back. At the time it seemed perfectly logical to me that if only we could get to the hospital quickly, via a helicopter, we could tell these idiots that our daughter was okay and that they were wrong. That's all I could think about. We had to get there RIGHT AWAY because we'd tell them they made a mistake, and we'd take our daughter home. It made sense. It was clear to me this was the only way it could be. I kept talking on and on about a helicopter, wondering who to call and how to arrange it. After hearing me babble for quite awhile, Alan said to me, in the most serious of voices, "THERE IS NO HELICOPTER." When I took in his words, and realized we had no choice but to continue driving, I started shaking uncontrollably. I couldn't breathe. I didn't want it to take four hours to get there in case they hadn't been doing anything for Jaclyn all that time. They thought she had died. In my head, I didn't believe this and wanted doctors to continue working to save her. Breathing was becoming more and more difficult for me, as the sobs grew more and more intense. At one point, Alan turned to look at me, pointed his finger in my face, and said, "If I have to pull over because you're not breathing, WE WON'T GET THERE!" I put my head between my knees and tried to contain the sobs and the shrieks and the moans that were coming out of my body ever so loudly and gutturally.

My Jaclyn. My beautiful Jaclyn. I don't know what I was thinking during that long car ride to the hospital. I don't remember much. It began to sink in at some point that our goodbye that morning, as we put three excited kids into a car for a fun day at the amusement park, would be our last to our daughter. I kept seeing her in my mind running toward me for a hug. I kept feeling her legs wrapped around my legs. I saw her waving goodbye as my cousin's car pulled out of the driveway.

I have no idea how we drove safely to that hospital. I don't know how Alan did it. I have very little recollection of the ride. I don't even know what time we finally got there. There was a sense of wanting to get there, but not wanting to get there. My husband and I were together, but in my own head, I was so alone as I walked through the door of that hospital.

There are parts of that night, and the many days that followed, that I can recall with the utmost clarity, every detail. Only now that it is after the fact can I describe it as if we were in slow motion. It didn't seem real that I was walking into a hospital to see my Jaclyn who, I had been told, had died. Eighteen months later I can say that a part of me really expected her to be fine when we walked into that room. We had been in hospital rooms so many times with this child, and she was always okay. How could this time be different?

Only hours before, I had been rocking on a bench in Michigan thinking about how fabulous my life was. In retrospect, it was the calm before the storm. How ironic. I had a husband who loved me. I had three amazing children whom I adored and who loved me unconditionally. And one of my children, in spite of chronic illness, didn't let events like nine surgeries in ten years, therapies, medicines, or medical equipment slow her down. Perfect life!

~ ~

It has been eighteen months since I kissed my Jaclyn goodbye. Eighteen months since I told her, face-to-face, that I love her. Eighteen months since she hugged me and almost knocked me over that August day. Eighteen months of not waking her each morning for school, not seeing her with a big smile when she'd come home from the end of her school day, not watching her dive into her homework, not playing games with her, not hearing her favorite music blare throughout the house, not hearing her sing, not seeing her dance through the family room, not hearing her say, "Goodnight, love ya, see ya in the morning" at bedtime. It has been eighteen months since my beautiful daughter walked through the halls of our house, slept in her bed, plunked down at the kitchen island for a quick game of *Hangman*, helped me cook, or laughed that infectious giggle that she had. It has been agonizing to live without her. And it will continue to be.

This one day took away all that Jaclyn and we had worked so hard at—keeping her healthy. There was simply nothing left that we could do. It was out of our hands. In one day, ten years of living, laughing, learning, and loving came to an end. She danced through life for ten years. And then one day her heart stopped. It just stopped, and despite having a pacemaker, her heart wouldn't receive the impulse from the device. It just stopped. One day.

Jaclyn's Journey: Lessons She Taught Me

When I began to write this book, Jaclyn was 9 ½ years old and thriving. She had not begun her round of four surgeries in four months yet, but she was doing well. I started the book because I felt proud of all she had been through in her life, always with that smile on her face and dance in her step. I felt it was time to tell her story because she was such an example of how to be triumphant in spite of illness!

Then her round of surgeries began, and yet I continued to write. I was more frightened of her surgeries at age 9 ½ than I was when she was younger. I've tried to understand that fear, but I'm not sure I can pinpoint it. Perhaps my fear was greater when Jaclyn was older because by then she was scared of surgery too. But it was more than that. I think, perhaps, as Jaclyn got older I simply knew her better and loved her more! The more I got to witness day after day who this phenomenal child was, the more I got to know the child that was Jaclyn, the more I loved her for who she was, and the more afraid I became of surgeries and what could go wrong.

But she came through those surgeries! Triumphant once again! There were more surgeries and hospitalizations than we had bargained for during early 2006, but she wrote notes to us while delirious and on a ventilator, sang her favorite songs in PSHU, and walked the hospital floors with IV poles in tow. What an inspiration! Then, after two surgeries in a week, one being an emergency, and twenty days in intensive care, she came home. Three weeks later, she performed a solo dance to a standing ovation at the school talent show. That summer she shone in all she did. She mastered tasks that had previously been impossible for her. She couldn't wait to begin fifth grade. She spent her last day, very excitedly, at an amusement park.

I began this book to be a gift to Jaclyn someday. I had wanted her to know her journey at some point, and especially how proud I was of her and all that she had overcome. It was supposed to be a book about her triumph, because as I was writing most of it, she was demonstrating everyday to me and the world that her life was truly a triumph.

But she wasn't supposed to die. This book was supposed to end on a different note. I had planned it to be a "Hooray for Jaclyn book!" It was meant to be a book to demonstrate how families *can* live with chronic illness, without the illness defining their lives. It was supposed to highlight how one can live with illness and still thrive, like Jaclyn did.

Over a year after she died, I wanted to finish the book as a tribute to her. But how could her dying be the end of a book that was supposed to be uplifting? The book was begun with the intention of ending happily. *Jaclyn can live, and can thrive, even in the face of illness, so others can too.* That was the original message I wanted to convey. This ending didn't fit. This ending wasn't okay.

Many friends have reminded me over the last eighteen months that Jaclyn's life **WAS** triumphant. She **DID** triumph over illness. For ten years she triumphed. My daughter danced through life for ten years, in spite of her medical condition! She tackled everything that was thrown her way—much of it unfair and scary—but she tackled it with a smile and a dance in her step. Always a dance in her step.

Ten years wasn't enough. It most certainly wasn't enough. I still have trouble accepting that her life was fulfilling despite being gone at age ten. I will never understand. I will never, never understand why her heart didn't grow the way it was supposed to grow. I will never, never understand why, after enduring all that she did, after enduring more than any adult or child should have to, that she didn't live a long life. The unfairness of that continues to torment me. I will never understand how she could be so fine one minute, and then so not-fine the next. But, given what she was given, a heart that didn't grow the way it was supposed to grow, my daughter did shine in the face of illness. She did not let things stand in the way of laughter, love, or a good time. She lived fully in her ten short years and shared a lot of love. She shared a lot of joy. And in her lifetime she taught me many things. It wasn't enough, but it was full. Yes, it was definitely full.

One of Jaclyn's favorite songs from *Wicked* was "Dancing Through Life." She listened to it all the time. And that's exactly what she did! She played. She laughed. Every single day she laughed. She challenged herself. She smiled. She made others smile. She taught. She cared. She thought. She questioned. She conquered. She learned. She shared. She created. She loved. Not a day went by in our lives that we didn't say "I love you" or that she didn't say it back. She inspired. She touched. And most of all she lived! Perhaps we had something to do with that as her parents. I tend to think it was just her way of being.

Dancing through life. That's the way Jaclyn did it. As painful, agonizing and unfair as it still is for me to live without her, I do believe that dancing through life is the way to do it! In the last eighteen months, I've been told by many that Jaclyn taught and inspired them too.

Now, this is a story for my sons, for Ryan and Joshua. It is a memoir of a sister they knew and loved—her story—a story they will have to hold onto as they dance through their own lives.

"Because we knew you, we have been changed for good." This is a line from another song in *Wicked* that now has such meaning for everyone who loved Jaclyn. Thank you, My Love, for teaching me and for teaching us. I'm so glad I got to be your mom. Dance through life. That's the only way.

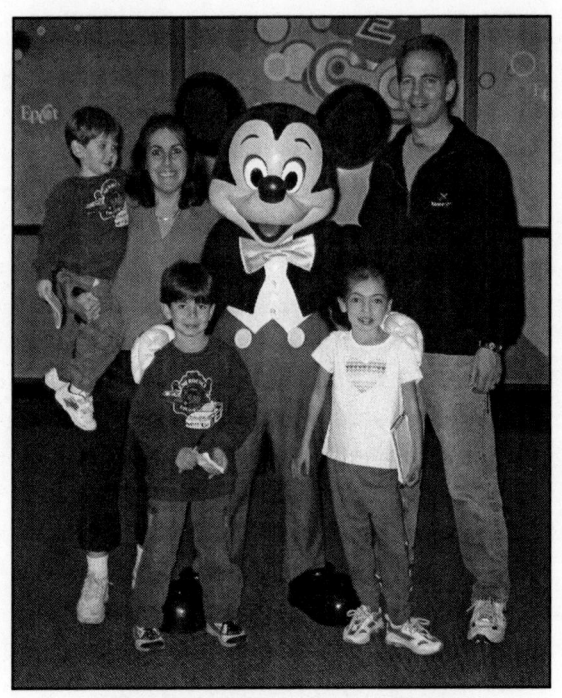

A family trip to Disneyworld.

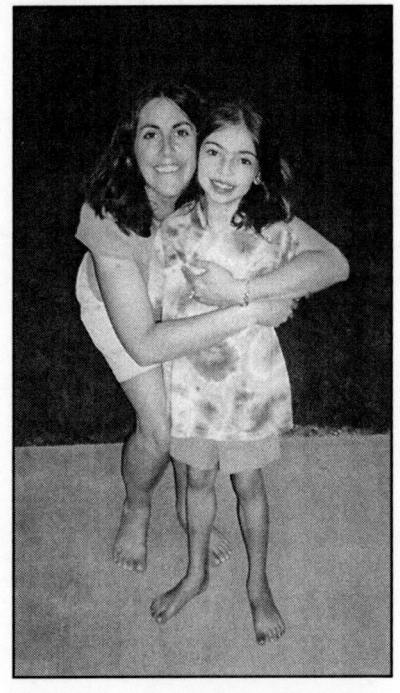

Jaclyn and Me together on a trip to Cleveland, June, 2006.

About the Author

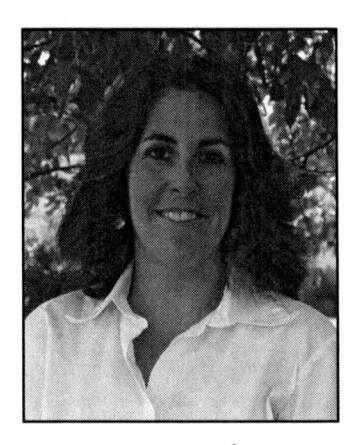

Lori Kaplan

    I married my high school sweetheart, Alan, after eight years of long-distance dating. I always dreamed of being a mom and of having a career as a college professor. Some of those dreams came true, but my perspective regarding what was really important changed over time.

    Today I am a stay-at-home mom who used to work as a Researcher and Lecturer. I have a Ph.D. from the University of Minnesota in Family Social Science, where I studied family relationships across the life cycle. I worked at the Rush Alzheimer's Disease Center in Chicago, studying the effects of Alzheimer's Disease on the marital relationship. My research was published in scholarly periodicals and presented at professional conferences. I also taught graduate level courses at the University of Chicago in the Department of Social Service Administration. Now that all seems like a lifetime ago.

    When Jaclyn was born, I traded in my professional hat to stay home and care for my daughter. I am also lucky to be mom to Ryan and Joshua who provide constant joy, laughter, and entertainment. Our three kids enjoyed a close, caring and affectionate relationship with each other. When we had to deal with upcoming surgeries or medical crises for Jaclyn, we met these challenges head on. But otherwise we tried to be a family like every other family - taking vacations, living our life, and having fun. Jaclyn wouldn't have wanted it any other way.

JaclynsJourney.com